Do you find yourself saying . . .

- I don't feel sick, but I don't feel really healthy either.
- Food is the most important thing in my life.
- I always feel hungry.
- I drink lots of cola to get me through the day.
- I *must* eat chocolate—or some other special treat—every day.
- Whether it's doughnuts, bread and cheese, beer, sweets, or junk food, I can't stop myself from bingeing on my favorite food.

No More Cravings

For centuries human cravings have been treated as a weakness or a lack of willpower, but in *No More Cravings*, Dr. Hunt demonstrates that hunger and appetite are part of a complex body system that requires stability and balance—and that cravings are often a result of metabolic imbalance. In this life-changing book, Dr. Hunt shows how your body may actually crave foods that you are allergic to—and how your health and happiness may be ruled by these uncontrollable cravings. Along with dozens of case histories, here are thorough, simple programs to help you find the causes of your individual cravings and end them safely and naturally—forever!

About the author

DOUGLAS HUNT, M.D., is America's foremost expert on food addiction. For over twenty years he has successfully treated more than fifty thousand patients suffering from allergies, hormone imbalances, phobias, and obesity. He earned his medical degree from the University of California at Irvine and is a member of the Orthomolecular Society, the International College of Applied Nutrition, the American Academy of Medical Preventics, and the Preventive Medicine Society. Dr. Hunt now heads a thriving private practice in the Los Angeles area that specializes in cravings. He recently hosted a weekly radio show, "Alive in L.A. with Dr. Hunt."

No More Cravings

DOUGLAS HUNT, M.D.

WARNER BOOKS

A Warner Communications Company

This publication contains various opinions of the author on nutritional subjects, which are stated pursuant to First Amendment guarantees for all writers and publishers. Any recommendations or opinions are strictly general in nature and should not be taken to apply to any given individual. The publisher and author, on their own behalf, wish to emphasize that the contents are intended to inform readers but are not intended to provide medical or nutritional advice for individuals, or for individual health problems. Such advice should be sought from physicians.

WARNER BOOKS EDITION

Copyright © 1987 by Douglas Hunt, M.D.

Cover design by Bill Graet
Cover photo by Simon Metz

Warner Books, Inc.
666 Fifth Avenue
New York, N.Y. 10103

 A Warner Communications Company

Printed in the United States of America

This book was originally published in hardcover by Warner Books.
First Printed in Paperback: March, 1988

10 9 8 7 6 5 4 3

To Mary, April, and Tina
whose love and encouragement have meant so much

ACKNOWLEDGMENTS

I owe a deep debt of gratitude to Denise Marcil, whose kindness and patience made this book possible.

A special appreciation to Beverly Trainer, the creative assistant everyone wishes he had.

Thanks to Fredda Isaacson for inspiring me to a higher level of professionalism.

Thanks also to all those other people who helped me in their own special ways: To Tamara, Anton Detric, and Bonnie, the girls and guys at the Hollywood Studio Typing Pool, and to editor and writer Lillian Rodberg, a strong upcoming talent.

CONTENTS

PREFACE

What is a craving? If you've ever made a midnight trip to the doughnut shop or driven out in a blizzard in a quest for cigarettes, you know how a craving feels, even if you can't define it. Since cravings involve substances that we take into the body in some way, we might call them consuming passions—desires so strong they can become obsessions.

Cravings are a signal of bodily imbalance

Anyone—young or old, fat or thin—can suffer from cravings. More often than not, what we crave are carbohydrates, usually sweets, but cravings for alcohol and drugs like cocaine have similar basic causes. They are related to the body's mechanisms for maintaining internal balance, or equilibrium.

Dr. Walter B. Cannon was one of the first researchers to explain how the body maintains equilibrium, a process he called *homeostasis*. The body has many automatic mechanisms for maintaining the most desirable balance of such factors as temperature, blood pressure, blood acidity (pH), and the levels of various substances needed to keep us alive and healthy. Pleasure and pain play important roles in driving us to obtain any substance our body needs. When we are deprived of the substance we feel pain or discomfort; when we obtain it we feel pleasure or a kind of relief that we may mistake for pleasure.

In other words, cravings basically are a signal from the body that homeostasis has been disrupted. Chemical imbalances are not all the same, and to eliminate the craving and restore good health we need to know what is missing or in oversupply. Cravings should never be ignored, for the underlying causes may lead to serious illness of body or mind.

Homeostasis: A complex process

What does the body consider a normal state, and what forces pull it out of balance? The human body is a marvel of complexity. For example, if the acidity of the blood rises even slightly, sensors in the brain activate the control centers for breathing. The lungs and the rest of the respiratory (breathing) system work faster to pump out the acid and restore normal balance.

A more striking, more easily observed balancing mechanism involves temperature control in warm-blooded animals. For humans, 98.6° Fahrenheit is normal, but this "normal" fluctuates, too. Our temperature tends to rise slightly in mid-afternoon and drop slightly in the early morning hours. Alcohol lowers body temperature; infections raise it. The body then strives to restore normal temperature, by increasing sweating to reduce a fever, for example, or by closing pores to conserve body heat. Our essential bodily processes function best at 98.6° F, so the body responds to changes in the environment in ways that maintain this temperature.

Homeostasis also applies to the mind

The concept of homeostasis applies to psychological as well as physical functions. Sensors throughout the body communicate its internal and external status to the brain. Any deviation from normal is immediately sensed by the brain, which must then decide how to respond. The human brain is a complicated network, though. Besides simple physical responses, it has stored within it all kinds of rules, fears, and behaviors. This super-complex computer, however, does not always communicate clearly; a simple message saying "send food" may emerge as a desire for a pepperoni pizza topped off by some chocolate eclairs.

Humans are the most complicated of animals. In pursuing the object of a craving we may be seeking taste pleasure, but we might also be yearning for the social contact that goes with a meal. We might skip eating to avoid gaining weight and then binge wildly in a kind of rebellious rage. Each individual has a repertoire of motivations for even the simplest acts. This human complexity can make it difficult to sort out the causes of cravings—yet conquering them is not as difficult as one might think.

Stress: The ultimate unbalancer

Homeostasis functions in three major areas: self-preservation, reproduction (species preservation), and stimulation (interaction with the environment). No individual or species can survive without some stimulation—yet too much stimulation, or the wrong kind of stimulation, produces stress, the ultimate unbalancer.

The body is continually counteracting stresses—physical, psychological, and social. If not handled properly, stress can lead to complete disorganization of body and mind. We humans are always at odds with ourselves: we need stimulation, yet our bodies need to maintain balance. When we seek stimulation, whether it is mental or physical, we come into contact with stressors that threaten homeostasis.

To handle these opposing forces we can use our *awareness*—the knowledge that experience and perception have given us. Unwise life choices often arise from lack of awareness. Yet men and women have always tended to resist awareness when they seek immediate pleasures that may lead to ultimate pain. Sometimes the very "badness" of the activity seems to enhance its momentary pleasure.

Many of our consuming passions lead us to seek substances that destroy homeostasis: tobacco, alcohol, caffeine, sugary foods, or various drugs. These substances disturb homeostasis and often lead to a destructive cycle in which the body's fight against the offending substance results in a feeling perceived as temporary relief—a mechanism I call *allergic addiction*. In this book these addictions are classified by type, but most are also in some way food-related.

Alcohol: A subject in itself

Cravings for alcohol and chemicals (drugs) deserve a book of their own. Alcoholism has been linked to a number of underlying causes, including hereditary (genetic) problems and problems of families and society. Yet serious food addictions are often found among alcoholics. Cravings for specific foods are especially likely to become obvious when an individual begins to abstain from alcohol. The nature of these addictions raises some interesting questions about whether alcoholics actually crave alcohol or the foods from which it is derived.

Beer and hard liquors are distilled from grains, especially corn, wheat, malt, and barley. Foods derived from corn are a major cause of allergic addiction, and wheat and malt are major allergens (allergy-causing substances), too. Wine and beer contain yeasts; cravings related to yeasts are especially severe. These are allergies we discuss in detail later in this book. Alcoholics who become abstinent often gain weight—often because of a greatly increased appetite for carbohydrates such as bread, pasta, and sugar. They need the "fix" they no longer get from liquor, and they need it in larger amounts. Liquor is metabolized (digested) more rapidly than food. Alcoholics who crave the quick fix they got from liquor may not be able to satisfy their cravings through food and will continue to crave alcohol.

On the other hand, alcoholics who have been successfully treated for food allergies report that their cravings for alcohol cease. Alleviating an underlying yeast infection often stops or reduces cravings for wine and beer. Nutritional supplementation for such aspects of alcoholism as hypoglycemia (low blood sugar), depression, anxiety, and lack of energy has added immeasurably to the success of the overall treatment. Nevertheless, counseling and group support are of paramount importance in recovery from alcohol addiction.

Conquering alcoholism requires strong commitment and a combination of therapies.

Cocaine and chemical takeover

Chemical addiction, too, is beyond the scope of this book, but since cocaine addiction is becoming an epidemic, a few words about it are in order here. Users of this and other drugs become destructively "hooked." The chemical appears to take over the body; the individual eventually is unable to concentrate on anything except how to get the next "rush." How does this happen?

We know that when a disease organism invades the body, it actively tries to take over. Its sole purpose is to survive and multiply at the expense of body cells. Cocaine and other addictive chemicals, though, are not living organisms. How, then, does their takeover occur?

A chemical gains its power by changing the chemistry of our cells in a way that alters the way we feel. Moods and emotions are compelling motivators; sometimes they are strong enough to overwhelm our awareness or survival instinct. Even knowing how destructive cocaine is for them, addicts eventually crave it more than life itself.

Cocaine addiction, like alcoholism, creates its own disease in susceptible individuals. As cells and tissues are damaged, the body tries to correct the damage. Deficiencies of the needed substances arise—perpetuating the cravings and worsening the imbalance. (We'll explain how this happens in a later chapter.) For example, researchers have demonstrated that the blood plasma of cocaine addicts is deficient in a chemical called tyrosine. When this and other deficiencies are corrected, the cravings for cocaine diminish or cease.

Substance abuse and deficient diet

The Aatron Company of Los Angeles, like similar firms elsewhere in the country, has been performing nutritional studies on drug addiction over a period of years. There is no doubt that the health problems of cocaine addicts and alcoholics are somehow related to the absence of general and specific nutrients in their diet. In experiments with animals, alcoholism has been "turned on and off" with simple changes in nutrition.

No one should attempt to treat any kind of chemical addiction without professional help and supportive therapy. For both chemical addiction and alcoholism, though, proper evaluation of the diet and correction of nutrient deficiencies is a significant part of rehabilitation. It should be done in conjunction with, not in place of, traditional therapies.

Homeostasis, stress, and disease

Our consuming passions can make us sick. Substance abuse, whether the substance is food or some chemical, leads to illness. If the problem is severe enough, and continues long enough—if the body is subjected to too much stress—permanent destructive changes can occur in our cells, our tissues, and our internal organs. Physicians call this *organic disease*. Consider this: The leading causes of death in this country are diet-related, including cancer, heart disease and stroke, diabetes, and hypertension (high blood pressure).

If body chemistry is disturbed but no cell damage has yet occurred, physicians call the problem *functional disease*. In this category are migraine headaches, insomnia, depression, allergy or hypersensitivity reactions, constipation or diarrhea, hypoglycemia (low blood sugar), heart palpitations, and premenstrual tension (PMS). To this list, add our consuming passions—cravings.

Cravings are not "all in your mind." They are physiological effects stemming from physiological causes that are explained in the rest of this book. Its purpose is to show you how to regain control over your cravings, your health, and your life. If you are like most victims of cravings, you have tried and been defeated not once but many times. Try again. In this book you'll find strategies that are easier and more effective than anything you've tried before.

PART ONE

What Are Cravings?

CHAPTER ONE

How It All Began

As my baby pictures show, I was fat soon after birth and stayed that way for a year or two. I was a waddling, Eskimo Pie–faced child, with bowling pins for arms and legs.

The lean years

When the Depression hit Oklahoma in the 1930s, my father lost his business. We lived in abject poverty. Days often passed without food in the house, and there were nights my sister and I cried ourselves to sleep without supper. Staying thin was not a problem to me in those lean days.

On Thanksgiving Day of my third year in grade school, my mother saved up enough pennies to buy us a box of Quaker Oats. A bowl of plain oatmeal mixed with warm water, without milk or sugar, comprised our Thanksgiving dinner.

At school the next day I was so gripped with stomach pains I asked my teacher to excuse me from class. She turned me over to the principal who, unaware of my starved condition, took one look at me and snorted: "I know what your problem is. You had too much Thanksgiving turkey yesterday, didn't you?"

All I could do was stare at the floor in silent humiliation.

She pointed an incriminating finger under my nose, shouting, "Admit it, you little glutton—you ate yourself sick! Now, didn't you?"

Too ashamed to tell her the truth, I mumbled feebly, "Yes, ma'am."

"I knew it!" the principal exclaimed over and over as she yanked me by the ear into the next room and promptly administered a sound spanking. Chastised and red-bottomed, I was sent home. But the spanking did nothing to relieve the distressing pangs in my empty belly.

By the time I reached preadolescence, the years of food deprivation had taken their toll: I was frail and skinny as a beanpole. I looked the way I felt: lean and hungry.

At the age of eleven I found a job setting pins in a bowling alley and earned 35¢ an hour to feed my family. The few spare pennies I saved for myself were spent on junk food. I could never get enough, particularly sweets. Every day after work I would dash over to the nearest soda fountain and guzzle down a half-dozen Coca-Colas in one sitting. Starved for the treats that I missed during the Depression, I quickly compensated for all those sugarless years. I was a boy obsessed, as much in body as in mind.

Because I was active in sports, I gained little or no weight in my preteens. YMCA outings, swimming, and hiking kept me a tall, lanky, 110-pound fourteen-year-old. As we used to say in the Dust Bowl, I was a "wiry little devil."

The U.S. Army changed all that. When I turned fifteen, I ran away from home and joined the service. There I discovered a gastronomical paradise. The accessibility of Army food in vast quantity converted me into a dedicated overeater. My favorite eating spa was the off-barracks USO hall where I would wolf down donut after donut. I took to the bottle—the Coke bottle. Fresh chocolate donuts and Coca-Cola became the deadly duo I could no longer live without. To me KP duty wasn't a chore, it was an opportunity.

Hooked on junk foods

I was *hooked*. I was a totally committed choco-cola junkie. And I gradually joined the ranks of the overweight. After I left the Army, I married a young woman with a penchant for potato casseroles, and with that my weight problem grew and grew. I ballooned out until I was *fifty pounds overweight*. The "Fatso" of my babyhood returned to haunt me, with the rotund face, bowling-pin arms, potbelly, and all. I became, in every sense of the word, obese. This up-and-down roller coaster effect can be seen in the histories of most overweight individuals.

But I was too young and naive to realize the seriousness of my problem. When I tried to lose a few pounds, it was impossible; I was too hungry most of the time. For even the most stout-hearted among us, prolonged physical hunger can be an unbearable experience. The average physician could offer nothing but useless advice.

In spite of my education, college and medical school, my obese condition did not change. After I was graduated and began my internship, it was necessary to spend long night hours in hospital wards. By this time I had a severe weight problem and had reached the point of awareness where I *knew* I had to do *something*.

I tried diet pills, with dire results. My body's system could not adjust to them, and I became a walking bundle of raw nerves. I fared poorly on the night ward. My mind couldn't function properly because I was too distracted by fits of nervous anxiety. Even when I stopped taking the pills, the internal warfare between hunger and crash diets was so overwhelming I could not think clearly.

One factor made the shedding of each pound a long, arduous task. It was something fundamental that took me eleven years to acknowledge: the *sugar factor*. Whenever I broke the diet on brief occasions, it was always with sugar or chocolate—and my weight would shoot right back up again.

"Big gulp"

Chocolate and cola continued to be a staple of my diet, and that was the real problem. My sugar cravings had reached their peak when I developed an addiction to Winchell's donuts and Pepsi-Cola in the "big gulp" size (from 16 ounces to half a gallon). I could not go home after work each day without bringing along at least a couple of these "big gulp" cartons. My wife would find empty containers scattered around the house—behind chairs, atop tall cabinets, under the bathroom sink, on the balcony ledge, in flowerpots, even in her sewing box. A visitor could walk in and literally stumble over a pile of cartons. Our home resembled a makeshift bottling factory.

Once my wife came home with an armful of "big gulp" Pepsis, and our neighbors asked whether she had some kind of mental problem. In fact, she did have a very serious problem: *me*.

The terrible realization finally dawned on me. My sugar cravings were wrecking my home life, my marriage, my body, my emotional stability, and my self-confidence. Every day or so I consumed up to a box of donuts and three or more "big gulps." My sugar fix seemed irreversible. When I drank colas I craved chocolate (a common phenomenon among sugar addicts, I have since discovered), so I always chased each swig with a mouthful of Winchell's best. The two were constantly associated in a vicious circle, as chronic and dangerous to my health as any heroin or cocaine habit. I was not only gaining weight, I was poisoning myself. It had to stop!

Cold turkey

Then I reached my second important decision: I must *never* eat chocolate or drink cola again, pure and simple. If I ever expected to have a lean, healthy body and start living like a normal human being, I had to kick the habit.

I tried to go cold turkey.

My first attempt was a disaster. In the course of only three days without sugar, I was driven nearly to a state of raving lunacy. I faced each morning with the firm conviction that this was the end of my addiction. By the middle of the afternoon, however, my cravings grew so overwhelming I couldn't stop myself—I lunged for that first donut and "big gulp."

At night I dreamt of chocolate. By day I entertained fantasies of owning a "big gulp" concession. Then, almost unconsciously, my car would veer toward the nearest 7-Eleven.

By the third afternoon I was in tears. I knew the day's battle would be lost again. I felt overpowered by my desire —helpless, abandoned of all hope.

From this experience I decided that willpower alone was not enough. My conviction and resolve knew no bounds, but to find the ultimate answer I had to open my mind to new scientific avenues of approach.

Psychology didn't help

This led to an in-depth study, not of the psychological roots of my cravings, but of possible biochemical causes. Considering that I had been a qualified expert on weight control for years and had treated thousands of patients, the odds were stacked in my favor. Or so one would expect. The fact was I had failed to cope with my problem despite my medical training, despite my special postgraduate interest in nutrition and weight control, and despite three years' training in psychiatry. Apparently, nothing I had learned up to this point had done me any good!

I decided to discard all I *thought* I knew and start from scratch. I had to rethink what obesity really was. Where do cravings originate? I intended to find out.

In my particular case, I had a severe physical addiction to sugar and chocolate. Some of you, reading this book, may be just as addicted; others of you may have cravings only once in a while. Regardless of the degree of your problem, this book can help you.

Character: Weak or strong?

We will be discussing theories about cravings in the next chapter, and then we will discuss the methods of stopping them. First, though, I want you to understand that cravings are *not symptoms of character weakness*. I bring this to your attention to discredit an old line of thinking that always leads to failure. That misconception is: "I will only be able to stop craving sugar or chocolate by strengthening my character.''

How many times have you heard: ''Get hold of yourself,'' ''You've got to make up your mind'' or ''When you want to badly enough, you'll do it''—all implying you aren't trying hard enough. Unfortunately, most people relate fatness to lack of character, so let's debunk that theory once and for all.

First, character is no more a property of thin people than it is of fat people. Anyone thin, fat, or in-between can have it or not have it. Obesity is *not* caused by lack of character.

Second, willpower, too, is no more a characteristic of thin people than it is of fat people. You either have it or you don't, and sometimes it varies in degree. It becomes a critical issue only if you happen to be genetically predisposed to obesity.

I want to make it clear that neither cravings nor fatness relate in any way to a lack in your personality. To illustrate this point, let's rethink together the actual differences between fat and thin individuals.

Willpower and appetite

In most cases, the hunger profile of the thin and fat are diametrically opposed. A group of patients once met in my office to discuss their weight problems. Two friends of the patients also participated, both of whom were thin. I turned to a slim, attractive young lady and asked the standard question:

''Can you eat anything you want and still keep your weight down?''

''Yes,'' she answered, as I expected. ''In fact, I can eat all I want. I can eat *anything* and not gain a pound.''

Then I asked an unexpected question.

''Are there any days when you *don't* feel like eating?''

She furrowed her brow in thought and replied, ''Once I went two weeks without feeling like eating much at all.''

My overweight patients were aghast. It had not occurred to them, as I pointed out, that there are more factors involved in appetite control than simply observing that thin people

DR. HUNT'S THIN/FAT PROFILE

<u>Thin People</u>	<u>Fat People</u>
Are often easily able to initiate activity.	Often feel too tired to do anything.
Have fluctuating appetites.	Have constant appetites.
Have decreased appetite under stress.	Have increased appetite under stress.
Have decreased appetite when tired or ill.	Have increased appetite when tired or ill.
Have decreased appetite when emotional.	Have increased appetite when emotional.

sometimes overeat. Most observers aren't around when thin people *don't* eat. My patients found it difficult to comprehend that, at times, *a lean person undereats* because of *lack of appetite*, and this compensates for the periods when that person overeats. Underweight people seem to be more "appestatically" regulated in their activity and eating patterns than the overweight.

The other outsider in my group, an attractive but pencil-thin woman, corroborated this. She recalled that, the day before, a very good friend had asked her in all seriousness: "When was the last time you ate?" She had to think before responding, "Oh my gosh, I haven't eaten since Sunday." She had fasted for nearly two-and-a-half days without even realizing it.

Again, disbelief rose from my overweight patients, all of whom knew precisely the last time they had eaten, right down to the minute. This woman who was excessively thin (though not to the point of anorexia nervosa) demonstrated one of the mechanisms that cause thin people to maintain their slimness.

A thin person usually loses appetite when he or she gets nervous or upset. Often even the thought of eating provokes nausea. The overweight, on the contrary, develop a tremendous increase in appetite during emotional crisis. They can't stop eating.

Psychologists often proclaim: "If you become nervous, your natural response will be to eat." This is true, however, only of the fat individual. And it is not just nervousness that provokes fat people to overeat—*any* emotion will do. If they are happy, they overeat. If they are angry, they overeat. In fact, the only emotion that can prevent overeating in the truly obese is stark, raving terror.

Different responses

It is not simply emotional triggers that make the difference between thin and fat persons, it is how each type reacts to those triggers. If the thin girl quarrels with her boyfriend, she feels ill at ease and can't stand the sight of food. If the overweight girl becomes upset with her boyfriend, she can't stay away from the refrigerator. If the thin child becomes sick, he doesn't want to eat. If the fat child becomes sick, unless nauseated, he usually wants to eat more. The thin businessman goes on a trip and often loses weight. The fat businessman does the same and often gains weight. If a period of overeating occurs in the life of a thin woman, she will soon lose her appetite and berate herself for overeating. If a fat woman overeats, she may be so stimulated by the food that she will go on a binge.

However, I must stress the fact that although obesity is *not* a psychological disease, it is true that there may be some psychological overlays, or secondary gains, from overeating. One cannot deny the pleasurable sensations that one receives when indulging, but this is the *benefit*, not the *cause*, of overeating.

All hunger is not the same

At the office group session I described earlier, one overweight lady volunteered: "My husband has so much willpower; this helps him stay thin. He gets hungry just like I do, but he's more able to control himself. The other day we were sitting at the table finishing supper, and I asked, 'Would you like dessert?' He said he was still a little hungry but didn't think he would have any dessert. Now *that's* willpower.''

Again, there's that myth: Fat people have less willpower than thin people. The real problem is neither the degree nor the intensity of willpower, but rather the degree or intensity of *hunger*.

Fat people, in actual fact, have more intense and frequent hunger than the thin person even though they often possess just as much, if not more, willpower. The difference is that the fat person and the thin person are not fighting the same battle. The thin husband appears to have willpower because he is warding off comparatively weak hunger. The fat wife appears to have less willpower because she is struggling against a more intense hunger. If, by some magic, the man acquired his wife's hunger level, we would see a man with less apparent willpower.

The "character factor"

The myth further suggests that fat people are lacking in character. This too is a ludicrous statement in view of history's roster of world leaders who had an abundance of "character" but were also overweight. National heroes such as Napoleon and Winston Churchill were, in fact, obese.

Overweight patients who come to my office complaining, "I just can't control myself! I can control almost every other part of my life, but I can't control my eating," are highly disciplined individuals who in no way demonstrate any weakness of character. Then, outside the office, I meet thin people who are totally undisciplined in every aspect of their lives, including their attitude toward eating. They seldom restrict their eating patterns, they eat everything the fat person eats, they eat the wrong foods, they overeat, and rarely do they show any sign of self-discipline. Yet they maintain their thinness. *The myth that thin people are thin because they eat correctly is an illogical absurdity that should be dispelled once and for all.*

Contrary to popular misconceptions, fat people often demonstrate more willpower than the thin person because they have to refrain from eating deliberately—an arduous task at best, whereas the thin person never has to practice such denial.

I must emphasize that this refers to the *naturally* thin and fat. It would not apply to a formerly fat person who is now making extraordinary efforts to remain slim. When you consider that 95 percent or more of those who lose weight gain it back within a year, you can see what a monumental task it is for fat people to reduce permanently. Those who do maintain their weight loss succeed only with great effort.

Just how or why do you get fat?

We do not know the exact physical causes for obesity. At present, there is no concrete scientific explanation why people regain their weight so readily, although researchers have come up with various explanations.

My experiences with thousands of patients have led me to these conclusions: First, there is an internal physical *need* for the body to regain weight. According to this "setpoint" theory, you don't regain weight because of carelessness, but because your body uses every available method to reaccumulate that fat. As an example, in the last few years, I have been seeing more and more cases of patients with previous intestinal bypass operations who are beginning to regain their weight. The pattern seems to be a gradual return of hunger, with particular cravings for high-calorie foods. In most patients, it begins four or six years after the bypass. The body seems to be duplicating the physical conditions that existed before the surgery. The body is relentless; it ingeniously finds ways to overcome every barrier we create.

The second reason why people rapidly regain their weight has to do with the food industry. There is an army of people (millions) whose careers and fortunes depend on your eating patterns. The more you eat, the more food you consume, the more money they make. If you eat enough for two people, someone's profits are doubled. Keeping people fed to the gills is big business.

Hundreds of millions of dollars a year are spent by the food industry to increase your consumption of food. Experts of all types—research scientists, motivational experts, psychologists, and marketing specialists—are hired by the thousands to devote eight hours a day, five days a week to finding ways to trigger your hunger and tingle your taste buds. You are the target, and if they can get you to eat, they've scored a bull's-eye.

Consider that your internal environment works *actively*, day and night, to get your weight up and keep it up, and then consider those professionals in the food industry who hire the best minds and spend millions of dollars to encourage you to be a big consumer. Now, is it any wonder if you lose the battle? You, the consumer, essentially unaware of advertising's subliminal influence, don't have much of a chance. So 95 to 98 percent of you who do manage to lose weight are doomed to regain it in a year.

Hunger: A relentless opponent

When a thin woman is hungry, but slightly distracted, she may continue with whatever she is doing for a while before she feels ready to eat. And if she has to prolong the wait, she can do so without much suffering. A thin woman may arise in the morning and eat or not eat. She may hurry through a busy day without lunch. If overtired at night, she may retire without dinner. This pattern could continue for more than a day if she is deeply involved with her activities. Now and then, thin people can last a day or so with very little food intake.

The opposite is true of the overweight woman. She may not wake up hungry in the morning, but as the day progresses, so does her hunger. It may reach extreme proportions by mid or late afternoon and become agonizing by bedtime. It is not easy to distract her when she is this hungry. She may become irritable, driven to eat simply in order to function.

A fat person cannot function as well without food as a thin person. There are thin people who do suffer intense hunger, but they are easily distracted from it, and often when they start eating, they are quickly satisfied. I have been around thin individuals who complain bitterly of hunger, but when they sit down to eat, they don't even finish their meal.

Certainly there are exceptions to the rule. But, after observing thousands of both thin and fat individuals throughout the world, I would submit my theories to any test with confidence.

The effects of aging

As we begin to age, most of us start to feel as if we possess less and less willpower as we experience more and more periods of overeating. In truth, we are not losing our willpower, we are developing an ever increasing hunger level. As people reach maturity, they apparently become more disciplined in every facet of life except this area, where they seem to weaken and lose power. This is not really the case, though. A mature person has *more* willpower than he or she did in youth; it's just that hunger becomes progressively stronger.

You won't find an explanation for this phenomenon in books. There is presently no scientific explanation why people seem to get hungrier as they get older, but it has been my observation that they do. I'm sure most readers of this book will agree. Not a day goes by that I don't hear a patient say that he or she notices how much harder it is to control the appetite—how it is definitely getting more difficult as time goes on.

I can testify to this myself. My hunger is more intense now than it was in my college years. I could say no to things then that I cannot resist now. I do not attribute this to a weakening of my willpower. Actually I am more productive and disciplined now than I was as a young man.

I used to say to myself: "The only interest I have in food is to survive. I don't really use it as a form of entertainment." Nowadays I say: "If I don't eat, if I miss a meal, I may be endangering my health.'' I fear the loss of a meal as though my life were at stake. My memory bank tells me, "If I don't eat, I'll suffer the penalty of foggy thinking or fatigue, if not actual pain." For me, missing a meal becomes a highly unpleasant experience.

When and how weight problems begin

Having helped more than 20,000 private and clinic patients reduce their weight has given me ample opportunity to ask them about the roots of their problem. Only a small percentage of them began life as fat babies. Many people have only a slight weight problem, or none at all, in their early years. But, as time passes, more and more break away from the norm and start gaining.

It is estimated that at least half the United States is either overweight or trying to reduce. Obesity has become a national problem, and what differentiates us from starving Third World societies is obvious: an abundance of food. Such plentitude, along with certain triggering agents, catalyzes obesity to a point where it is virtually irreversible.

Before this "triggering" has propelled you into obesity, your body regulates itself automatically. However, once you have been triggered into actual obesity, you must exert conscious effort to maintain control. You are forced to switch from automatic to manual. And the change in your response to foods and the change in your eating patterns follow. Take, for example, the case of Mrs. Smith:

"Mrs. Smith, last year, before you had your baby, did you overeat when you got nervous?"

"No."

"Do you overeat now when you get nervous?"

"Yes."

"Did you seem to have more willpower a year or two ago?"

"Yes, but since I have had my baby, I seem to have lost it."

Not until this interview was Mrs. Smith aware of the change in her response to foods.

As time progresses from the triggering period to a current level of obesity, overweight persons often forget what they were like when they were thin. I have seen this in thousands of cases: The pattern is predictable, and yet the personalities of those who undergo this change vary greatly, indicating to me that personality has nothing to do with becoming obese.

Common trigger mechanisms of obesity in women include pregnancy (most likely the first baby), birth control pills, emotional shock, severe illness, and certainly many surgical procedures such as hysterectomies. I have seen thousands of women who gained weight after a hysterectomy, despite promises from their doctors that it would not happen. In later life, of course, menopause frequently steers the aging female toward obesity.

In men, the major trigger mechanisms of obesity are an end to the smoking habit, sudden job changes with a decrease in activity levels (such as a promotion from workman to foreman), and often alcohol. Since it is virtually pure sugar, alcohol is often a major contributor to weight problems, as well as being a strong appetite stimulant.

The stairstep effect

A critical factor related to obesity is that it can gradually increase owing to aging or from successive traumas to the body. For example, a woman may gain twenty pounds after her first baby, another twenty after an emotional shock, then another score at menopause. She may go up and down a number of times in the interim, but each shock to the body tends to upset its delicate balance and prevent it from returning to its previous norm.

The balance necessary to maintain thinness gradually erodes and is lost. Obesity is basically a stairstep disease: You may lose twenty pounds, then gain it back plus another ten; then you may drop that thirty pounds, but your next gain is another thirty pounds plus ten or fifteen more. There seems to be an overshoot effect each time a person regains his weight.

The 300-pound man you see walking down the street was not born obese. In fact, he may be able to show you pictures of himself as an underweight young man. Slowly, over the years his body changed, and he found it extremely difficult to stay down.

Overeating overworks all organs of the body. The heart must pump more blood to the tissues, often two or more times the norm in a grossly overweight individual. The digestive system is overloaded. The amount of insulin necessary to accommodate this extra load can be so great that the pancreas cannot produce sufficient insulin, that is, the person develops diabetes. Eighty percent of all people who develop adult-onset diabetes develop the disease when they are rapidly gaining weight. It is a severe stress on the body when foods are poured into it continuously.

Every time you gain or lose weight, you send shock waves through your body similar to those produced by an operation, an emotional shock, or sudden change in lifestyle. It is there-fore important for the overweight person to realize that he or she must stop stairstepping large amounts of weight because this in itself contributes to the worsening of the disease.

"Hidden" hunger

Another phenomenon related to the overweight, and one that often confounds us, is *hidden hunger*. A certain percentage of overweight people will claim they are not really hungry, but they seem to feel like eating; or they say that though they feel no hunger, they eat continuously because of nervousness.

Hidden hunger is physiological in nature. The overweight man or woman frequently has a poor connection between the brain, the stomach, and other organs that feed back the in-formation that produces hunger. In other words, such people do not know when they really *are* hungry. When tubes with gastric balloons to record contractions were inserted into the stomachs of a group of thin people, it was found that as their stomachs contracted, their brains registered sensations of hun-ger. From this it was concluded that if thin people feel hunger, it is directly related to actual physical need.

When the same experiment was performed on obese in-dividuals, the findings were different. Sometimes they complained of hunger when there were no simultaneous stomach contractions. At other times, there were recorded contractions, but the obese individual did not feel any conscious hunger. This makes it difficult for obese people to control their eating. Their conscious feelings of hunger do not in any way correspond to their bodies' needs. They may know they have eaten enough for their daily supply of nutrition, yet they still feel they should eat more and feel endangered if they don't.

Another part of the hidden hunger syndrome that is even more maddening occurs with people who *never* receive the signal that they are hungry. In other words, there are hunger contractions in the stomach, but never a light on the switchboard. They *feel like eating*, even if they don't feel *hungry* —because they have no idea whether they are physically hungry or not. This is often expressed as "I never feel hungry, yet I want to eat all the time."

This common but not easily recognizable malady may be similar to a disease called *dysponesis*, a condition in which the brain confuses signals from different parts of the body. It is often seen in the syndrome of referred pain, in which one may register a pain sensation from an area where there is no pathological disturbance or tissue damage. The equivalent hunger confusion can present insurmountable problems for those who are overweight.

Physical versus mental

There are many *physiological* differences between the fat person and the thin person, but most of them are *results* of obesity, not causes. But—and this is the important point to remember—there is no conclusive evidence of any *psychological* difference between fat and thin persons that can be directly attributed to their appetite problems.

If you have only a telephone relationship with someone, and you're not allowed to question him about his weight or eating habits, what question could you ask that would tell you whether or not that person is overweight? None, of course. In fiction, fat people are often characterized as lazy or jolly, but in the real world these same traits could be just as easily applied to thin people.

My contention is that, in most cases, obesity is not a psychological condition but a disease derived from the disturbed physiology of the human body with some psychological overlays.

For fifty years and more, we have been bombarded by endless publications and articles by psychologists on how to control weight. No doubt you have read some of them. Have they in any way aided you in curtailing your weight gain or in stopping your cravings? If not, why not? Simply because *your problem is not psychological*. No amount of advice about oral fixations, stroking behavior, game playing, or any other psychological theory has had any real effect—certainly not in my own experiences with 20,000 patients. The fact that at least 95 percent of Americans who lose weight regain it within one year has not changed in the past half century. If "weight psychology" worked, we would be a nation of slim, self-controlled individuals, not a land of wall-to-wall fatties who are gaining new pounds every year.

Behavior modification: Fat chance!

Behavior modification has been recently promoted as the new answer to obesity. There has been a continual flood of articles to publicize its success. I have, however, heard it criticized at medical conventions, and I have seen thousands of failures. Psychologists have adopted the view that they can condition, train, or even brainwash a person into maintaining a particular psychological reorientation related to weight control. In fact, no amount of reorientation under clinical conditions is effective enough to stand up to the outside world. A person may go through a "training" program to lose weight and stay down, but, upon reentering society, that person is quickly deprogrammed by the food industry and reoriented to eating the way he or she did before.

I regard behavior modification as a popular medical and psychological fad that will have its day until it is eventually supplanted by more realistic treatments for obesity. The well-informed today believe that new physiological and pharma-cological techniques will arrive in the not too distant future. Some are already looming on the medical horizon.

Discarding the psychological approach: The real solution

If the psychological approach to craving and hunger control is incorrect, what other facts can be applied? *Experiments with animals have demonstrated that there is a relationship between cravings and nutritional deficiency.*

If I had never experienced the problem myself, and if I had not decided to stop beating my head against the wall, using accepted but useless medical techniques, I would not have found the new approach that is presented in this book. What I learned in my search for the real cause of obesity and cravings is that the psychological approach is bankrupt, and the physiological approach is the only one that will work.

CHAPTER TWO

What Are Cravings?

A search of medical literature reveals little reference to cravings. In a similar search of psychological literature, we find cravings listed under appetite. Appetite is believed by most professionals to be due to psychological causes. The *American Heritage Dictionary of the English Language** offers the following definitions.

> *Appetite*: 1. a desire for food or drink 2. any physical craving or desire 3. a strong wish or urge to partake of something 4. to strive after, desire eagerly. [Most young doctors are taught that hunger is physically felt, while appetite is learned and is mostly psychological.]
> *Hunger*: 1. a strong desire for food 2. the weakness, debilitation or pain caused by a prolonged lack of food 3. mild discomfort or uneasy sensation caused by lack of food 4. a strong desire or craving for anything.
> *Crave*: 1. to have an intense desire for 2. to need urgently; require 3. to beg earnestly for; implore.

*(New College Edition, William Morris, editor, The Houghton Mifflin Company, Boston, 1976. Used by permission.)

> *Craving*: 1. a consuming desire, longing or yearning.

Dictionaries usually represent current thinking of the public, and these overlapping, confusing definitions are probably what most people believe. A precise definition is not so important, but it is necessary that you as a reader understand what I am talking about when I refer to cravings.

What I describe in this chapter is *actual physical dependency on certain foods*. It's easy to understand how this condition could develop from drug use, but how does it work with food? It is likely the same process exists in both situations. I will describe one theory of how this happens later on. It is my belief that physical dependency can develop as a consequence of a substance-created deficiency.

Nutritional deficiencies

First, how do deficiencies develop in our overfed society? There are many explanations. For example, it's easy to understand malnutrition in elderly persons who have made unwise food selections. Note how cafeterias catering to this clientele always place dessert first in the line of foods. This is done to encourage the patron to build the meal around the final treat. Studies in gerontology indicate that many senior citizens have multiple nutritional deficiencies.

Following World War II, Japan was inundated with imported sugar. The Japanese went wild. An explosion of vitamin B deficiencies was documented, caused by excessive sugar intake. This experience put an end to the belief that if you eat good food along with a lot of sugar, you will still be well nourished. Large amounts of vitamins and minerals are needed to metabolize excessive sugars, thus making one vulnerable to deficiencies.

Heavy use of alcohol falls into the same category as overuse of sugars. Alcohol becomes pure sugar in the body and requires large amounts of vitamins and minerals for digestion and excretion. Sugar is sugar, whatever its form, including the "acceptable" forms of sugar, such as fruit juices. In other words, *large amounts of natural sugars in rapidly absorbable forms are just as harmful as artificially made sugar.*

Another cause of deficiencies is consumption of large amounts of caffeine-containing beverages such as coffee, tea, or diet drinks. Besides caffeine, these fluids contain other chemicals that must be metabolized as well, such as phosphorus, which affects mineral balances and requires body responses to retain normality. But the most serious problem that arises from overuse of these beverages is the diuretic effect. Excessive fluid loss flushes out large amounts of water-soluble vitamins and minerals, creating deficiencies.

Drugs commonly used in medicine also put demands on body nutrition. A good example is birth control pills, which cause a number of vitamin shortages. A medical journal recently reported the results of a study on the use of diuretics in heart disease patients. It indicated an 80 percent higher rate of death in those taking so-called water pills. Well-informed nutritionists blame this on chronic mineral depletion.

Disease, of course, can put huge demands on the body's store of nutrients. After an episode of flu, many people report the development of cravings and an intense hunger.

Street drugs such as marijuana are notorious for creating the "munchies" (cravings) following usage. I've treated these munchies as deficiencies, and I've been quite successful.

Stress and emotions are also triggers for hunger and cravings in the obese and even in individuals with normal weight. Hundreds of experiments have documented the rapid intake of nutrients by organs busily manufacturing the various necessary hormones and chemicals that must assist the body's response to stress. One hour of rage in a schizophrenic can use up thousands of milligrams of vitamin C. The thinking process itself does not use extra calories or extra vitamins and minerals. Emotions especially when they are intense, *do* burn up additional calories and nutrients, because they increase the heart rate and other body functions.

Some nutritionists believe that a woman seeking the proper amount of vitamins and minerals from food would need a daily intake of 3,500 calories, which is about what the average woman required at the turn of the century; but now, of course, the average female only uses about 2,200 calories a day. To "eat right," she would have to become overweight. The only solution is to take supplements, but only a small percentage of our society does that regularly. So, if the above theories are true, then most people are running the risk of at least borderline deficiencies.

Ivory tower nutritionists claim that deficiencies don't exist in our society, and they quote computer data to "prove" it. I don't agree with them. I see patients every day with symptoms of deficiencies that respond to vitamins and minerals.

Cravings in animals

I know of no conclusive medical research on why people crave items such as chocolate, sugar, and colas. But there have been studies on other cravings, especially in animals. We can easily relate these findings to sugar cravings.

In a recently published book, *The Hunger for Salt* (Springer, 1982), we find comparisons relevant to most cravings that affect us. Salt cravings are well known to farmers and ranchers who raise domestic animals, as well as to veterinarians who attend these animals. Reports of these cravings have existed for centuries. Man, along with the animal kingdom, has also been a seeker of salt. The commercial and economic development of many societies has, to some degree, revolved around the availability of salt. It was once transported by gigantic caravans of camels in both Asia and Africa to the great salt markets of the ancients. This commerce was later to give way to sugar markets.

Salt is the principal mineral of the body and is of vital importance to good biochemical balance. Humans and animals seek it because it is necessary for survival. A famous axiom of allergists is, "The only thing the body absolutely cannot become allergic to is salt." The absence of salt can cause great concern and can quickly motivate a lot of effort to obtain it. Humans and animals will always spend whatever time is necessary to maintain their supply. Strangely, even though we all know we need salt, the exact mechanism that motivates us to seek it is still in the realm of theory.

From the study of salt cravings, we can reasonably assume

that the body has built-in hunger symptoms for the intake of all components it needs. In addition to salt, animals are known to develop a craving for bones, which contain phosphorus. Cattle and wild game grazing on phosphate-deficient pastures have been reported to eat bones. These reports have come from various parts of the world over the past two centuries.

It's been well established that such behavior is associated with low concentrations of phosphorus in the blood. Research scientists have long been aware of such cravings and are continuing the search for answers. They are interested in knowing just how an animal chooses the right food. What we do know is that when a creature is deprived for some time, specific drives are engendered by the state of deficiency.

How does the animal determine that it needs a particular substance? This too is the subject of ongoing scientific investigations. *Certainly the greater relief provided, in answer to the urgent need, the more addicting the substance becomes.* (When does a craving become an addiction?)

Experiments with cattle who were known to be phosphorus deficient showed they had a specific appetite for bird feces or newly ground bone. This appetite disappeared when phosphate was injected. In other words, as soon as the animals in this experiment got what their bodies needed, they stopped eating bird feces. As soon as *your* body gets what it really needs (the materials recommended in this book to block the cravings), you lose your appetite (cravings) for foods that are not good for you—sugar, chocolate, and colas.

Blood levels of calcium and phosphates have a definite influence on feeding behavior; Scott (1950) showed that calcium-deficient rats had a preference for high-calcium diets. After removal of the parathyroid gland (parathyroidectomy), their calcium intake increased to as much as thirteen times the normal levels but returned to normal with treatment. Calcium-deficient chickens, in one report, ate eggshells constantly. Calcium-deficient pigs were noticed, in one study, to lick the lime from the walls of their cages.

Other deficiencies also affect eating behavior. Pigs found deficient in vitamin A were seen to search diligently for a blade of grass or weed that might come through a crack in the floor. There are numerous experiments indicating that a

pica = strange cravings

mineral deficiency causes the animal to have cravings for the missing ingredient. Magnesium and potassium deficiencies also showed some relationship to special food selection. In relationship to the behavior of cravings and appetite, the self-regulatory capacities in animals is a relevant but still comparatively unexplored area.

"Strange" cravings

One of the oddest examples of "strange" cravings is called *pica*. Pica is an appetite perversion that provokes the ingestion of strange or unsuitable or even repulsive substances. *Pica* is the Greek word for magpie, a bird known to eat unusual objects. The phenomenon occurs throughout the world and has been recorded for centuries. The most common explanation is that those who evidence pica are seeking trace minerals or inorganic minerals missing from and desperately needed by their bodies.

The disease is seen in many animals—cows have sometimes been observed eating nails and wire and rusty iron objects, and cats have been known to eat ashes and charcoal. In cases reported in current medical literature, the substances most commonly ingested are dirt, coal, clay, chalk, starch, pebbles, wood, plaster, paint, soot, hair, and cloth.

Eating is not the only way substances are ingested. There is a case on record of a woman who for days on end breathed in the odor of musty books. (A yeast-allergic individual could possibly receive a "high" from breathing in the odor and the spores of mold in the books.) Many women report severe hunger when they cook dinner and smell the aroma of the food. Vapors are merely airborne solids and often cause the same reaction in the body as the original substance would have, had it been eaten. One patient was found to be addicted to breathing in the odor of old shoes. Still another patient ate woolen and leather garments, and an older man with pica ate rodents' nests complete with dead and live mice.

In the 1930s and 1940s a familiar comedy theme involved a pregnant wife who wakes her husband up in the middle of the night to complain of wanting ice cream and pickles or

Pagophagia = ice craving

some other unusual combination of foods. The strange cravings experienced by pregnant women are universally acknowledged. Some have been known to request salty or acid foods, but others require more exotic items such as oyster shells or ashes.

Pagophagia, or the craving for ice, is rather common and is often seen as a sign of anemia. One of my recent patients had severe chronic anemia and constant cravings for ice. She always carried a cup with her. This type of anemia, associated with ice craving, is known to be hereditary.

In the lab

Vitamin deficiencies also cause specific selection of foods in laboratory animals. Whereas salt is specifically recognized as a separate entity by animals and humans that lack it, *vitamin B and other vitamins are far less specifically recognized. They are hard to identify and do not create specific appetites, for they do not occur in an isolated fashion in nature.*

Cullen and Scarborough (1969) have shown that normal rats with a marked preference for sugar over salt reversed their eating patterns when they were made salt deficient. There is abundant evidence to indicate that laboratory animals value sugar highly and will endure pain in order to get it. This does not necessarily indicate sugar deficiency; it may result from habituation or addiction.

Cannibalism, or who's for dinner?

Believe it or not, cannibalism by choice (cannibalism, famine, and hunger are covered later in the book) is believed by some scientists to be motivated by a search for minerals. The Amazon Basin with its enormous rainfall is of particular interest in this respect because the regional natives have a very low salt intake. The area is also suspected to be low in calcium and phosphorus. Endocannibalism (eating relatives or tribal members) is or was practiced there, particularly the consumption of the ground-up bones of the relatives. The bone powder is added to *caxire*, an alcoholic beverage. Bone consumption may be a recycling of minerals, which are deficient in that area. It is possible the practice was first initiated under circumstances of extreme deprivation, producing a substantial sense of well-being and thereby combining an organic need with symbolic ritualism. Cannibalism is apparently an ancient practice. Broken skulls from prehistoric man reveal that in some cases human brains had been extracted for consumption. In Peking, Neanderthal, and Cro-Magnon man, the same evidence exists; e.g., the Neanderthal skulls found in Java may have been opened in this manner.

Instances of cannibalism have also been reported in early Europe and Ireland. Marco Polo and other travelers reported Chinese and Tibetan tribes eating the flesh of fellows. Colonies of termites and other insects have been turned into cannibals by creating mineral deficiencies. Cannibalism has been reported in hyenas, who eat their own young, and in wild chimpanzees, lions, sharks, and other species.

Indian tribes of the Northwest Pacific ate flesh "for the gods." The human sacrifices of the Aztecs are well known. Similar sacrifices occurred in Fiji, Central Africa, and New Guinea. The most striking example of cannibalism in recent times, however, occurred in 1970 when an airliner crashed in the Andes Mountains of South America. Young survivors existed by eating the bodies of the crash victims. From descriptions of how they selected blood clots from around the heart, scientists suggested that their bodies sought out the minerals and, most important, the salt found in the blood. They ate in obedience to their cravings, to maintain the minimal nourishment for survival. Of course, cannibalism has existed for a variety of reasons; deficiencies are only one of many motivations.

Something is missing

The basic hypothesis of my program is that *cravings are physical and not psychological*. The triggering event prior to the cravings may be psychological in origin, it may be stress related, or it may be related to the actual development of some dietary deficiency. The end result is a vitamin and/or mineral deficiency. The missing minerals or vitamins, when returned to the body, stop the cravings.

These deficiencies, whether they are actual or relative (minerals tied up and unavailable), result in the development of unpleasant symptoms and the need to seek relief by seeking out specific foods.

It is important to note here that the human body, and nature in general, are *not* always wise. The body can be fooled by counterfeit substances that in some way relieve the symptoms of a deficiency without supplying the needed missing ingredients. Counterfeit substances behave in the following manner:

1. They relieve the unpleasant symptoms of a deficiency.
2. They create a greater deficiency in the process.

Withdrawal symptoms

Let's use cocaine as an example. When cocaine is ingested, by any method, it poisons the organism. The affected person will have to metabolize poisons as quickly as possible. To do this, the body must mobilize large amounts of vitamins and minerals from its reserves. This mobilization of reserves creates a lot of energy in the body which gives the individual a mood elevation, that sought-after "high." The individual undergoing this unusual energy gain (albeit a false one) assumes the experience was good because it produced pleasure. (Pleasure centers in the brain are also stimulated.) Later, when the cocaine (the toxin) is totally exhausted, the individual experiences an energy loss, because so much of the protective material was used in a short period. What was intended to be used up over a period of days was expended in hours. Even with supplies short, the individual must continue to function normally, to breathe, to have heartbeats, to move, and so on. The body will try to redistribute nutritional supplies. But this, obviously, leaves all the organs deprived. The person then develops symptoms of not feeling "right"—to put it mildly.

As an example of one function: The blood pressure may have risen when the person took cocaine and experienced mood elevation, but without the support of all that extra energy from metabolizing the cocaine, and with the resultant lack of energy to support the blood pressure, it begins to drop. The body, in danger of losing consciousness, quickly releases adrenaline (epinephrine). This burst of adrenaline into the bloodstream causes shaking hands, nervousness, anger, impatience, and moodiness—in a word, withdrawal symptoms.

Withdrawal symptoms can occur with any toxic substance, whether it's cocaine, coffee, or nicotine. Even food substances such as sugar can become toxic in excessive amounts. Substances to which the body is allergic acutely stress it; they act like toxins, cause the body to overreact, and use up large supplies of nutrients.

The individual who is coming down off a high has unpleasant sensations ranging from mild uneasiness to total panic, depending on the amount of toxins ingested and the amount of materials used up in the body's attempt to detoxify itself. The individual then begins to crave relief. The question then becomes, *what* does that person turn to for relief? *Here is where the body confuses itself, and the addictive process begins* (whether it be to drugs or to food).

The body has chosen the wrong path. It may not have enough sensitivity to correct its mistakes. It is, therefore, up to the mind to produce an answer. There are endless examples in nature where animal instincts and innate wisdom are not sufficiently developed to produce the proper responses.

When deficiencies occur there is a need to restore vitamin and mineral balance, but the body does not necessarily interpret the need correctly. If only a single major mineral is missing, such as salt, the internal information feedback systems make it clear to the brain that salt will bring relief. Ample research in this area makes it undeniable that salt cravings relate to salt deficiencies. However, when there are *multiple* deficiencies of less clearly defined vitamins and minerals, messages to the brain are often confused. The brain cannot get a clear picture of what substance would relieve the discomfort. Individuals then crave symptom relief rather than a cure. They think that cocaine made them feel better, so they try it again and, sure enough, they *do* feel better—in fact, they feel wonderful. It worked; they achieved the sought-after relief. They are unaware that their bodies must scramble again, borrowing from Peter to pay Paul, and must again mobilize all possible reserves from other organs and systems to get rid of the toxins that represent danger to the tissue. Once again these individuals experience the pleasurable effects of all that energy. Of course, in time, they will need larger amounts, because the body won't be able to respond to lesser doses. There are additional physical explanations for the development of drug dependency, but I have emphasized only what I consider to be similarities between food and drug addictions.

The October 1984 issue of *Psychiatric Annals*, in an article entitled "Psychopharmacology of Cocaine," reports a test of 26 vitamin deficiencies in 26 cocaine abusers. The findings are summarized in Table 1. The report states in part:

> . . . The tremendous electrical discharge [by the cells] seen during cocaine use makes it necessary that [certain] vitamins be supplied to the [central nervous system] in sufficient quantities.
>
> In an effort to learn more about the effects of chronic cocaine abuse on catecholamine and indolamine precursor and vitamin co-factor levels, we undertook a pilot study in which we analyzed the vitamin profiles of 26 cocaine-abusing individuals on admission to Fair Oaks Hospital. . . . The vitamins tested included Vitamins A, B_1 (Thiamine), B_2 (Riboflavin), B_3 (Niacin), B_6 (Pyridoxine), B_{12}, C (Ascorbic acid), and folate. The amino acids tyrosine and tryptophan were also measured.
>
> Nineteen of 26 (73%) individuals had at least one vitamin deficiency. . . . These results suggest that cocaine abuse is associated with multiple deficiencies, principally Vitamin B_6 (Pyridoxine), B_1 (Thiamine), Vitamin C, and tyrosine. These deficiencies may be specific to the cocaine abuse or may be a result of malnutrition since cocaine is an anorexic

Table 1
VITAMIN DEFICIENCIES FOUND IN
26 COCAINE ABUSERS
(Data from *Psychiatric Annals* 14:10/October 1984)

Vitamin or Precursor	No. (%) Below Normal	No. (%) Above Normal
At least one	19 (73)	5 (25)
B_6 (Pyridoxine)	10 (40)	——
B_1 (Thiamine)	7 (28)	——
C (Ascorbic acid)	6 (21)	——
B_2 (Riboflavin)	6 (21)	——
B_3 (Niacin)	——	——
B_{12}	——	——
Folate	——	——
Tyrosine	7 (28)	——
Tryptophan	——	——
Vitamin A	1 (.4)	5 (25)

agent and severe cocaine abusers tend to ignore all bodily needs including eating. Metabolic considerations may also be important since Vitamin C is a co-factor of tyrosine hydroxylase, the rate limiting enzyme of norepinephrine synthesis. The high Vitamin A levels may be due to high levels of Vitamin A found in raw cocaine.

Our findings suggest that patients with cocaine abuse should be evaluated for vitamin deficiencies. Treatment of those amino acid and co-factor deficiencies helps stabilize the patients' medical status and makes them more amenable to treatment of their cocaine abuse.

Short-circuiting the cycle

My approach to cravings is to replace the missing vitamins and minerals during the craving phase and thus short-circuit the cycle. If the right vitamins and minerals are supplied to the body, the cravings simply disappear, because there are no symptoms to deal with.

Finding the *correct* minerals and vitamins is the key, because each substance is metabolized in a slightly different way. Some drugs, for example, are eliminated from the system through the liver, some through the kidneys, some through the lungs, others through the skin, and so on.

If I give a patient who has sugar cravings an intramuscular injection of minerals, that person stops craving, usually within 10 minutes, and the cravings do not return for five to ten days. I've done this thousands of times and have found it works 100 percent effectively. Minerals given orally may potentiate one another, and it is these combinations that I deal with in the book, because everyone will get a different response.

While my focus has been on sugar and related food cravings largely ignored by scientists, other cravings of a more serious nature, such as the craving for salt, have been richly researched, and these results support my hypotheses. In the past, cravings in humans have been ignored or dismissed as a nuisance complaint. But solving the problem of cravings may solve a myriad of other conditions simultaneously. It's time to take cravings seriously and to provide help for those who suffer from them.

PART TWO

Quick Control of Your Cravings

CHAPTER THREE

How to Control Cravings for Chocolate and Sweets

Even if you crave sweets, chocolate, or colas only occasionally, you'll be helped by the supplements suggested in this chapter. And if you're a person who salivates at the mere thought of a Hershey bar or a cola, you'll find the formulas that much more rewarding. Whatever the degree or frequency of your cravings, read on. Help is on the way.

What about "that time of the month"?

If you crave chocolate, sugar, or Cokes just before your period, and only at that time, you can learn how to control those cravings with the program presented in this chapter, plus the material on premenstrual syndrome found in Chapter 11.

What about other types of cravings?

Many people who think they have a weakness only for sweets often reply when asked what kind of goodies they prefer, "Oh, cookies, toast and jam, breakfast rolls, and I also love Mexican food, pasta, all kinds of bread and cheese." Well, if that describes you, Chapter 4 covers additional cravings in more detail, so read this chapter and the next one and combine both strategies.

If your cravings zigzag back and forth from sweets to salt, or if you crave other types of foods, read this chapter first. Then turn to Chapters 5 and 6.

You are one of a kind

It would be wonderful if the body possessed a chemical simplicity so that craving control would be as simple as buying a tee shirt where one size fits all. But physical chemistry is complex, and no single supplement suits everyone. Fortunately, however, most of us can get results quickly by selecting the supplements that best fit our profile.

To receive full benefit from the methods described, you must understand that the conditions related to the intensity, duration, and type of your cravings are subject to change. You'll need to learn about biochemical individuality in relation to the "average dose." In addition, stress and other related conditions may require your changing your supplements as you go along. And finally, timing, adverse reactions, and self-defeating behavior are important factors. Although these may sound like a lot to consider, don't worry. By applying common sense and using careful observation you can find the individual program suited to your needs. In the next few pages, you'll begin to see the whole picture.

The nutritional approach:
Is it more effective than psychology?

Yes, definitely. But to understand why, we must explain the difference between the causal mechanism of a craving and the "trigger" that sets it off. When you flip on a light switch, the switch itself has nothing to do with the light. It merely allows the electrical current to travel to the bulb. Electricity, not the switch, caused the light to go on. The biochemical processes behind our cravings are simply turned on by a switch or a trigger. Unfortunately many people, professionals included, often mistake the switch for the underlying chemical imbalances. These imbalances are usually a result of:

1. Food allergies
2. Vitamin and/or mineral deficiencies.

Psychological factors can switch on the "current" that causes the cravings, but so can a lot of other things. It really doesn't matter which triggers cause the chemical imbalance. *The ultimate need of the individual is simply to restore the balance*. The choice then becomes, "Will I use nutritional supplements, which can do the job in 10 or 15 minutes, or should I spend time and money on a psychiatrist's couch?"

Although one might, in fact, be able to rebalance disturbed biochemistry through psychological techniques, the effort and time necessary to do so are enormous and often not practical. Self-hypnosis can sometimes be effective, but one can't always conjure up a trance at moment's notice. Self-imagery, relaxation techniques, and biofeedback can work, but these also take time and conscious effort. Worst of all, however, these techniques often fail. If you decide to "make" them work, your level of success will depend on the time and effort you are able to invest.

All things considered, the simpler solution is to ingest a readily available natural substance, which can resolve the problem of a chemical or food-allergic imbalance within a few short minutes with no struggle at all on your part.

There's no such thing as an "average" person

The first thing to understand about this method, if it is to work effectively for you, is the concept of *biochemical individuality*. This simply means that no one human being can really be considered "average." Each individual's internal chemistry is as varied and distinct as his or her fingerprints.

Though our external appearances adhere to a pattern, internally there may be wide differences and deviations from the norm. Each of us has two eyes, one nose, and one mouth, and yet none of us looks exactly like the others. A broad range of important variations distinguish real people from the hypothetical "average person." This is true of every parameter, ranging from anatomy, biochemistry, and neurology to psychology.

Anatomical studies of the normal stomach, for example, have revealed hundreds of significant variations. The size, contours, and content of the stomach are incredibly diverse. When the Mayo Clinic studied the gastric juices from the stomachs of thousands of healthy adults, the level of the digestive substance pepsin, as well as the level of hydrochloric acid, were found to vary 100- to 200-fold.

In another study, a group of apparently healthy adults were studied for the levels of three different carbohydrate-splitting enzymes present. The results revealed a 10- to 20-fold variation in the quantities of enzymes present.

It is important to know that each person has a distinctive internal environment all his or her own. The list of nutrients needed may be the same, but the *amounts* we need differ. In addition, the way we handle these individual nutrients also varies. Even genetically identical twins show some variation in their biochemistry, and these differences can be surprisingly great.

When nineteen individuals were studied for their calcium needs, for example, the range of normal need varied from 222 to 1018 milligrams (mg) per day. The difference between the two extremes is 1 to 4.5. This is a significant difference between seemingly normal daily nutritional needs. And when the individual's lifestyle changes radically, of course nutrient needs may stray even farther from the norm.

Vitamin C, B_6, B_{12}, and D requirements have all been proved to vary widely from one person to another, and these findings will likely carry over to almost every known nutrient. Our inborn individuality has an undeniable biological basis. Evolution itself could not have taken place if this individuality didn't exist. In fact, the speed at which evolution takes place may be determined by this propensity toward individuality.

The fallacy of the "average dose"

In preparing pharmaceutical medications before the advent of pill stamping and encapsulating machines, physicians ground herbs into fine powders in crucibles, placed them in envelopes, and handed an envelope of powder to the patient. The instructions recommended a starting dose, then suggested: "Take as much of the medicine as necessary to relieve the symptoms." Today, people would perhaps react more favorably to medications if they were prescribed individually rather than on an average-dose basis.

An important axiom of nutrition states that whereas one person may not be harmed by a given substance, another might be; conversely, what may be ample amounts of a given element for one person might be completely inadequate for another. You cannot determine your nutritional requirements according to those of your neighbor or relative, or even from the advice of a medical authority. You can determine it only by your own experience.

The stress factor, or conditions that change the dose (such as the changing intensity of the cravings)

As you work out your own requirements for nutritional supplements, remember to take into consideration *all* of the conditions that exist in your life at the time you experience your cravings. For women, normal physiological conditions that may alter the body's requirements include pregnancy, hormonal changes prior to menstruation (PMS), and menopause.

The whole gamut of life's trials and tragedies ranging from death and divorce to lesser life adjustments exert different levels of stress and strain on the individual. You must decide for yourself in each stress situation whether you need to increase or decrease the amount of the supplements you are using.

Consider your own psychological make-up: How have you adapted to stressful events? Some people react stoically to a crisis, calm on the outside but tense on the inside. Others tend to dramatize each experience, consciously acting out every emotion. However we react to stress—and reactions vary according to time and situation—its effects can be minimized by making sure we keep our physical chemistry in balance.

Timing the treatment *take before they become intense)*

It is important to know that each dose of a nutritional supplement will last only a limited time. The prescription I administer to myself and to my patients usually lasts between four and five hours, but this, too, varies from person to person. In severe stress situations the dose may have to be repeated every one or two hours. On the other hand, some individuals may need only one dose per day.

For the first day or two, you should make a conscious effort to keep track of the time when the dosage seems to wear off and your cravings begin to return. Once you have determined a schedule, you can then easily continue the pattern.

To determine the dosage necessary for a premenstrual craving, you could use the technique described above; the dosage will probably be the same in subsequent months unless your symptoms vary in intensity. The same dosage can be used also before ovulation. Many women forget that ovulation, which occurs halfway between menstrual periods, is another time when strong cravings can occur. For more detailed instructions on how to deal with these special problems, read Chapter 11.

I must also encourage you to be patient. If your first attempt to stop cravings does not succeed, adjust the amount of the supplement and the length of time between doses.

Another point about timing: Once you know the amount of materials that keeps your craving under control, you must alert yourself to the very first signs and symptoms of the craving and take the medication *before* they become intense. The longer you wait, the less effective the supplements will be.

Let me demonstrate why this point is so important. If you were to consult a psychologist about a problem, such as uncontrollable outbursts of anger, he or she would probably teach you methods of handling the problem. He would probably advise you to become aware of the earliest beginnings of your anger so you can take corrective steps before it becomes so intense that nothing will control it.

The problem is, people are so often unaware of the early changes in their moods that the mood reaches an uncontrollable level before it's fully recognized. The sooner you become aware of your cravings and take action, the more likely you are to be successful.

How strong are your cravings?

Supplementation is varied according to the intensity of the craving: mild, moderate, or severe. If your problem is mild, you may crave sweets, chocolate, and colas only once in a while, perhaps several times a month. The cravings may only last a few hours; the longest period of time would be a day. Your cravings might last only until you get the desired candy or cookie—then fade and not return for days. We'll call this Category One. Here you can use one or two supplements *very* successfully.

An example of Category Two would be the cravings women get prior to menstruation. The cravings are moderately strong—intense enough to cause weight gain, but not necessarily severe. These women may also crave sweets at other times of the month, and the craving may last for days. This category of patient is probably addicted to sugars, and yet Category Two people usually do not identify themselves with physical dependency or addiction.

Category Three people are slaves to their addictions; their cravings for sweets or chocolate are frequent, intense, and often related to emotions. These people are under much self-imposed pressure and frequently overreact to their problems. They say they use food to calm themselves and to escape unpleasant feelings. In this group you will find those cravers who drink colas virtually all day long, just as coffee addicts drink coffee.

Before thyroid test - no kelp for 2 weeks

A word of caution on possible adverse reactions to the supplements listed

1. If you are allergic to iodine, it is important that you test the Min-tran (below) carefully and don't take any form of iodide.
2. If you are about to have your thyroid checked, you should not take kelp for two weeks before the test.
3. If you've ever experienced adverse reactions to *any* of the items listed below, do *not* take them. Look instead to other chapters for help.

Almost any individual without a very severe health problem may take this formula without fear. Keep in mind, however, that anyone can be allergic to any substance. If you develop a rash or itching, a headache, or general aches and pains, stop taking the substance, then switch to another form of the same substance after those symptoms have disappeared. You still may be able to get craving relief from another similar product.

When the cravings start, what then?

The sooner you start your craving control, the smaller the supplement dosage required. As an example, when I first notice a patient just beginning to crave sweets, I have that patient take two Min-tran tablets with a large glass of water, every three hours during the day and especially in the evening. Min-tran is a broad spectrum mineral formula with extra calcium. If you are allergic to iodine, be cautious about this or any supplement containing iodine, including kelp. If the cravings are not too intense, one or two days of this routine is enough. Add two additional tablets to the first two if the cravings reappear, but this higher dosage should not be taken regularly.

If the craving for sweets is rather strong I suggest the patient take four or more tablets with a large glass of water every three hours for several days. Obviously, the dosage and frequency of usage depend on the intensity of the cravings. It's important to keep the neutralizing effect going continuously, especially during the first day or two. I've found doses at three-hour intervals to be about the best schedule for most patients. After the cravings begin to fade, usually in one to three days, the regular schedule may be discontinued and the supplements used only when needed. *Note:* Patients with premenstrual syndrome (PMS) may have to adhere to a tight schedule to control cravings for the entire week or so of premenstrual cravings (see Chapter 11).

Most people report immediate relief after the first dose and total relief after the second dose. It is vitally important that the doses be taken consistently to keep the cravings fully suppressed. Taking the pills now and then will not give the desired results. Often when patients report they aren't being helped by the treatment, we question them and find they simply are not taking their minerals properly.

Almost everyone can tell within 30 minutes to an hour whether the substances are working effectively. But let's say you've not experienced relief after conscientiously trying the supplements for a day. Now I add a second substance. In addition to two tablets of Min-tran I tell the patient to take three or four 3000 mg tablets of desiccated liver with a large glass of water every three hours. In my experience, Min-tran alone has stopped the cravings of more than half my patients, but adding liver tablets has significantly increased the success rate. You have noticed, I'm sure, I didn't say 100 percent. There are some hard-core cravers who require something more to block their biochemical imbalance.

I have found Min-tran to be the best starting material for cravings, but it is often difficult to purchase except through the manufacturer's outlets or pharmacies. You may call or write Standard Process Laboratories, 2023 West Wisconsin Avenue, Milwaukee, Wisconsin 53201, for sources in your neighborhood.

Let's say you can't find these items locally and you need something more readily available. You may wish to start with a combination of kelp tablets (150 micrograms) and calcium lactate (5 grams). Three tablets of each, with a large glass of water every three hours will do the work of the Min-tran. As mentioned before, keep the schedule up for two days, then use the supplements only as needed. If you are careful not to eat the craved foods carelessly while in the midst of the cravings, the cravings will surface less and less often.

Kelp tablets usually have a maximum of about 150 micrograms (mcg) of iodine; most manufacturers make about the same strength tablet. Just read the labels and take the strongest one you can find. Liver tablets contain about 3000 mg. Read the labels and use the strongest one. Calcium lactate tablets are usually available in 100 to 500 mg tablets. I often recommend Lilly's 5 grain (324 mg) tablets, which most drugstores carry. The stronger the tablets, the fewer you need for craving relief. Experiment to find the fewest tablets that are effective. So far I have not found a kelp-calcium tablet, but if you find one, use it in place of the two separate items.

Sometimes the supplements fail to work because, unbeknownst to the patient, the gastrointestinal tract is not breaking down and absorbing the tablets. I have seen more than one X-ray study showing intact, undissolved supplements near the end of the patient's bowel. Along with this, patients report seeing undissolved supplements in the stool. Since the supplements cannot work when they are not absorbed, I take an alternative approach in these cases. I suggest that the patient take one tablespoon of *liquid* calcium every three hours along with the kelp and a large glass of water.

One of the most effective combinations I have found is three tablets of kelp and three calcium lactate tablets taken with an aspirin (sodium salicylate) and a large glass of water every three hours. After several days of this regimen, as-needed usage is suggested. Inexpensive 10 grain (650 mg) aspirin tablets can be purchased at any pharmacy. One to three aspirin a day is safe for almost everyone. Larger dosages should be limited to two-day periods only. Do not take aspirin if you are allergic or sensitive to it, and remember that long-term, frequent usage of aspirin can produce a large number of dangerous side effects. Fortunately most people have good commonsense and know when they are using too many. So far these easy instructions have not caused anyone harm. Some manufacturers recommend a maximum of eight tablets a day. Aspirin is very useful in helping to combat cravings, but it should be used judiciously. I haven't found Tylenol to be quite so effective.

A kelp-calcium-baking soda combination can also be effective. Use one teaspoonful of baking soda in a large glass of water along with three calcium lactate tablets and three kelp tablets every three hours. An Alka-Seltzer Gold tablet can substitute for the baking soda. Use one in a large glass of water. Baking soda tablets are also available at most pharmacies. Three of these tablets can be taken with the kelp and calcium combination.

This regimen may seem like a lot of pills to take, but keep in mind that not as many pills may be needed for every individual and that this dosage level is for several days only and for just occasional usage afterwards. The minimum dose that will work is my motto.

Category One people will usually get relief from the preceding combinations, but now let's tackle the more difficult cases. If you are in Category Two, you may need more oil. The essential fatty acids make minerals more available to the cells and thus more readily utilized by the body. There are both fast and slow ways to get results.

The fastest way I know to get almost 100 percent success, if there are no other underlying problems, is to use Complex F tablets from Standard Process Laboratories in addition to calcium lactate and kelp. The essential fatty acids found in Complex F act on the cell walls to aid calcium diffusion. They help restore the balance of the involuntary nervous system. This combination, besides stopping cravings, may also function as a natural tranquilizer. Four to six Complex F tablets together with three calcium lactate and three kelp tablets usually stop cravings immediately. If Complex F tablets are not easy to obtain, substitute essential fatty acid capsules, linseed oil capsules, or cod liver oil capsules. Three capsules of any one of these along with the three kelp and three calcium lactate tablets should be swallowed with a large glass of water every three hours for several days. All the oil capsules contain about the same amount of linoleic, oleic, and lenolenic acid. A final boost for the basic calcium-kelp formula is L-glutamine, an amino acid that helps raise blood sugar. Take three 500 mg tablets in addition to the previously recommended combinations.

A slower but excellent way to gain control of cravings for sweets or colas is to adopt a routine of taking three evening primrose oil capsules, 400 units (IU) vitamin E, and 400 micrograms (mcg) of selenium daily for at least three months. If this works for you, you can continue this regimen indefinitely because it is a healthful one. Use the various combinations of kelp and calcium in conjunction as directed. As you notice these formulas becoming increasingly more effective, you may find you require fewer supplements to do the job.

Dr. Robert S. London of the North Charles General Hospital has reported that use of vitamin E alone, over a period of several months, reduced craving for carbohydrates and particular sweets. The essential fatty acids and selenium make vitamin E more effective, so there should definitely be some benefit to this program. Category Two people should have their cravings under control by this time.

People whose cravings do not respond to the above programs usually have mixed cravings (they crave multiple foods such as sugar, colas, bakery products, and salt) or they have serious underlying health problems. Those with multiple food cravings will need the additional supplements suggested in other chapters of the book. All cravings must be treated simultaneously because each individual craving serves as a trigger to other cravings.

Any underlying health problem that may be causing cravings must be treated, or the cravings will persist. Hypoglycemia (low blood sugar), hormone imbalances, digestive difficulties, food allergies and mucocutaneous candidiasis are some of the diseases that may cause cravings. These subjects are addressed later in the book. Category Three people, those with underlying diseases, are crippled by their cravings and unfortunately the foods they overindulge in contribute to their underlying disease. Their cravings may be caused by the disease, but controlling the cravings is essential to the treatment of the disease. Although self-help is always a good idea, it only goes so far. Unrelenting cases may require professional help, sources of which are listed in the last chapter.

How long can you take these supplements?

Can you use this formula indefinitely with the objective of permanently blocking the craving impulses? The answer to that should be no. It probably would be better if you used the formula intermittently rather than continuously, although I see no harm in continuous use for a few months. Prolonged use, however, might cause you to become unresponsive to the effects of the supplements, for the body changes its response to substances if exposed to them for too long.

An ounce of prevention

Another successful approach is to use the formula in a preventive way—that is, starting the formula several days before the expected cravings. The cravings that occur before a menstrual period would be a good example. Each month you might begin the formula three days before you anticipate the onset of premenstrual symptoms. That way you can prevent the cravings before they have a chance to take hold.

The body: A rebel without a cause

Some people wait too long to begin taking the supplements, and this is often a case of unconscious rebellion. Once you have reached a certain level of discomfort, your body will seek immediate gratification. For example, if you are forced by some social circumstance to hold your bladder for a long time before urinating, you undergo a great deal of discomfort, which may be expressed by a tightening of your muscles. When relief finally comes, it is so pleasurable that you actually enjoy the experience of releasing the painful muscular tensions. A good deal of pleasure can be had when a strong pain is suddenly relieved. The same kind of response can occur with cravings.

Take the case of the man who was addicted to baking soda. Apparently when he had gas and took baking soda, it caused him to belch. The relief obtained from the release of gas was so pleasurable that he deliberately took anything he could to create bubbles of stomach gas so that he could relieve the tension and obtain more pleasure.

If you allow the cravings to build up to too high a level, the desire to rebel against anything that will block the enjoyable relief of your symptoms will be so great that, even if you have the supplements on hand, you may ignore them and choose to fulfill the craving for the sheer pleasure of it. Relief from high tension can be in itself addicting in a self-destructive way. Thus it is important to get the cravings before they get you.

Skepticism: Did it really work?

One of the most common reactions to the successful blocking of a craving is doubt and skepticism. So often I've heard the comment, "Well, my cravings have stopped, but I don't know whether it's the minerals or if I just psyched myself into thinking they worked." In our society, we are so oversold on the idea that everything begins and ends in the mind that when a physical solution is effective, we tend to doubt the results. Of course you can easily test the prescription by taking it and then not taking it. In this way you can observe how the cravings come and go and can recognize that they only stop for good when you use the minerals. If you stay on your program properly and conscientiously, you will have the control you've always wanted.

Inconsistencies

Another common resistance to using the formula properly comes from the fear that taking vitamins or minerals in large amounts can be detrimental to your health. Let me give you an analogy. Some patients feel they should take antibiotics only if they have symptoms. So they take less medication than is prescribed and then stop taking it altogether the instant their symptoms disappear. They fail to understand that an absence of symptoms does not necessarily imply the defeat of disease. It only indicates that the disease is in remission, while the original infection could very well still be present.

This timid approach to the proper use of medication tends to thwart its effect and prolong the problem. It allows the bacterial strain to familiarize itself with the antibiotic and thus develop an immunity to it, sometimes causing greater complications in the future. The best way to use any medication is full strength in the beginning, as prescribed, and not a single dose fewer than directed.

Twelve additional suggestions for craving control

The following suggestions were taken from medical literature. Some of them may also help relieve your cravings.

1. Self-control method. The principle here is that you crave sugar because you were conditioned to want it from childhood. You can't eradicate a sweet tooth, but you can control it. You must first recognize your obligation to deal with the problem, then be *willing* to deal with it and believe that you can do it. In other words, take responsibility for your own actions. No one else puts food in your mouth. It is *your* hand that reaches for that candy box on the table. You must take positive steps to change this behavior.

    a. Start out by completely avoiding the items you are craving. Don't go near them. Get them out of your own environment totally, and avoid restaurants if they cause temptation.

    b. Accept the fact that this is not going to be a picnic. You may have withdrawal symptoms, so expect them, and be prepared to handle them.

    c. Choose substitute foods whenever you get a craving. Try fruit, cherries, grapes, even a baked apple with cinnamon. You can relearn your habits if you work at it.

    d. Resist that first bite. The longer you stay away from sweets, the more the tendency decreases, until finally you free yourself of the desire. Always keep in mind that, as with alcoholism, the first drink will start the whole process going again.

The basis of this treatment is that you will think and plan your way out of the problem. You will not say to yourself "I need a donut." Instead, you will say, "I would like to have a donut, but I don't really need it." The supposition here is that intellect conquers feelings.

People live through their hearts, not their heads. Sugar traps you emotionally and physically rather than intellectually. This technique will work but you must be very conscientious.

2. _Exercise and small snacks_. This idea suggests a regimen of eating every two hours along with a regular program of exercise. You are warned that you must take responsibility for the condition of your health. This approach prevents your blood sugar from becoming too low (hypoglycemia) by encouraging frequent meals. The theory is that your blood sugar will be maintained at a level high enough to keep you from getting caught up in the craving syndrome.

This constant eating can prove to be more damaging to weight problems than helpful, so choose your foods carefully. If you use this method, you must be very conscientious. If you get careless and miss a meal, back will come your cravings. And you start all over again.

3. _Sugar cutdown method_. "Gradually reduce your sugar intake" is the message here. As suggested by Nathan Pritikin's diet book, _Lose Weight Feel Great_, you use two teaspoons of sugar in your coffee instead of your usual three and continue to slowly reduce the dosage, thereby weaning yourself off the culprit sweet.

The danger here is that even a small amount of sugar may just prime the pump for wanting more. Some of my patients have stopped craving sweets this way; but they were not severe cases. You will definitely need the supplements also.

4. _Creative sublimation method_. This method recommends involving yourself in creative pursuits. Every time you desire

sweets, you indulge in your hobby and use this as a pleasant substitute for the desire to eat sugar. Be aware, though, that unless you have carefully selected a very interesting or highly recreational hobby, it won't stand up against a trip down to the ice cream parlor. It can't just be a good hobby, it's got to be a *great* hobby. You'll need a careful plan to make this method successful.

5. *Cold turkey method.* You begin by gathering everything in your home that has sugar in it, then tossing it in the trash. (And don't forget to take the garbage out. You might change your mind later.) If this creates deficiencies in your household supplies, then you go out and buy sugarless products. In this way, if you start to break down, you have nothing within reaching distance to satisfy the old desire. If you can't get your hands on it, then you can't get it into your mouth to perpetuate the craving.

6. *Sugar substitutes method.* Here you are asked to try substituting natural sweeteners such as honey for table sugar. Then when you have weaned yourself off sugar, you gradually wean yourself off honey or at least keep it down to a minimum. You're supposed to keep lots of records of what you eat. Then if a sugar cop asks you for proof, you have plenty of documentation. Seriously, if you require sugar in your coffee, then cut out the coffee. Switch to tea, plain or with honey. This approach is not unreasonable, but you must work on it diligently.

7. *Lemon in water method.* The idea here is that lemon juice will acidify your body fluids and tend to drive out the cravings for sugar. This is partially beneficial at times. We have another method to stop the cravings by changing the acid base balance. You'll read about it in Chapter 5.

8. *Magnesium method.* Take 300 mg magnesium three times a day, evenly spaced. This is an old trick used by bariatric physicians. I use magnesium as a supplementary aid, and it is sometimes useful. Many doctors have suggested it to their patients and have reported some success. You might want to give it a try. Use 300 mg tablets in the chelated form.

9. Water method. This is the advice of several self-help diet books: Drink at least ten glasses of water a day, and as many noncalorie carbonated beverages as you wish. Bloat yourself with water so that you have no room for cravings. A variation of this technique is to alternate glasses of warm and cold water.

Since water runs through the stomach very quickly, the effect is only transient. Alternating one glass of hot water and one glass of cold water does confuse the stomach enough to diminish hunger sensations, but the result is only temporary. Remember to stay close to a bathroom.

10. Bile salts method. A well-known nutritionist suggests using double dosages of bile salts during cravings. I have not found this very helpful, but you might want to give it a try. You can buy bile salts in health food stores. It can't do any harm. It's been used by some physicians successfully. I have more to say about this in a later part of the book when we discuss digestive enzymes.

11. The permission statement method. Instead of *commanding* yourself not to eat, you give yourself *permission* not to eat. For example, if you enter a market and pass the irresistible chocolate cupcakes, you do not say to yourself: "I am going to pass this by" or "I had better not buy that or I will start eating again." Rather, you tell yourself: "I have permission to take good care of myself. I have permission to pass this by and still feel great. I can walk by here and be totally happy that I said no to this food."

You may notice that you can sometimes pass desserts by without difficulty, though some people would argue with that. Here is what usually happens: If you use a *command statement*, you may stop yourself from picking up the cupcakes at that moment, but you'll likely be fantasizing about them while you dutifully push your cart over to the diet section. By the time you're in the check-out line, you're likely to be so aroused that you make an eleventh-hour dash back to the cupcakes. So much for commands. A *permission statement* tends to relieve you of this tension and might eliminate that self-destructive rebound.

I have had some success with the permission statement, but although it can be effective, most people probably won't use this technique for longer than about a week. If you want it to work for you, make sure you keep it up until it becomes a habit. If you forget to use it often, you will eventually abandon it altogether.

I have suggested this technique to patients who were conscientious enough to try it. When they reported back within a day or two, they would tell me how effective it was. A week or two later I would query them, and they would snap their fingers and say, "Oh, yeah, you know, somehow or another I got out of the habit and forgot to use it." Regrettably, the benefits of the permission statement are strictly short-term unless you make a resolution to use it until it becomes a deeply ingrained habit.

12. Positive and negative imagery method. Stand in front of the mirror and talk to yourself. Examine your appearance and what it could become. If you are not terribly overweight, imagine that you have become quite fat. Or, conversely, see yourself in a beauty contest wearing a bathing suit and ask yourself how you'd rate. See yourself naked in a crowd and wonder what people would think. If you'd rather look on the bright side, imagine yourself as thin, and *staying thin*, when you have cravings.

As good as this technique is, it can be psychologically painful. But then that's the idea—making it too difficult to eat the wrong things. It's a good method if you do it often enough to form a habit. And it helps to have good mirrors.

The last word

Some of the preceding twelve methods may also help you with your other cravings, especially if you apply them seriously. I used some of them for years.

These methods can be used in conjunction with the mineral supplements. However, they may be unnecessary. You should probably reread the first part of this chapter to be sure you understand craving control before you read the next few chapters and gather ideas for your own personal program.

CHAPTER FOUR

How to Stop Craving Bakery and Cheese Products

When I first treated people who complained of sugar and chocolate cravings, I assumed that a cookie craving was the same as craving for a chocolate bar. After all, a sweet is a sweet—or is it? Some patients responded favorably to the treatment, but others did not.

A cookie craving is not a sugar craving

Because of some failures with the previous formula, it was necessary to question the patients more carefully about the types of food they were attracted to. A pattern gradually emerged. Some patients were attracted to candy and sugar per se, while others were attracted more to sugary bakery products such as cookies, donuts, rolls, pies, cakes, or pastry. By the use of an allergy-testing technique, I was able to determine that bread and cheese cravers were allergically addicted to yeast and wheat; those craving sugar were more susceptible to corn, and chocoholics were affected by cocoa. Later I learned there was still another reason for craving breads and cheeses; that reason is discussed later on in the chapter on yeast infections.

The more patients I questioned, the more I realized that

gaining weight from foods containing yeast was very common. Actually, more people craved and gained weight from bread and cheese than from sugar. I had to rethink my methods to treat yeast and wheat cravings effectively.

Is allergy the culprit?

Although I'll cover masked or hidden addictions as a cause of cravings in the chapter on allergies, I have a few words of comment here.

Usually patients don't consider food allergy as a source of their problems, for food allergies are hard to detect. Allergic reaction to the food isn't always as obvious as a rash or runny nose. It's more likely to cause the highs and lows connected with physical dependency, as well as painful withdrawal symptoms. Food addictions differ from drug addiction only in degree of severity.

The most commonly eaten foods are the ones we're most likely to become addicted to, and yeast-containing foods certainly fall into that category. If the food is eaten more often than once every three days, an allergy may develop. For example, most people eat yeast daily in the form of toast, sandwiches, and so forth. Wheat is also commonly ingested (see box). It, too, can be responsible for cravings. Milk is another product in bakery goods that can trigger problems. We'll later explore just how yeast infections are a cause of bread and cheese cravings.

FOODS THAT CONTAIN YEASTS, MOLDS, AND FERMENTS

DEFINITION

Any substance which is derived from, cross-reactive with, or contains in either substantial or trace amounts: yeasts (sometimes called leavening), molds (also called fungi), ferments (processes of souring, fermentation, fermentation hydrolysis).

SOURCES

1. Substances which contain yeast, molds, or ferments as basic ingredients.

ALL RAISED DOUGHS: Breads, prepared "ice box" or frozen breads, and biscuits.

ALL VINEGARS: Apple, distilled, wine, grape, pear, etc. This includes all foods containing any vinegar, e.g., salad dressings, mayonnaise, pickles, catsup, sauerkraut, olives, most condiments, sauces such as barbecue, tomato, chili, green pepper sauces, mince pie preparations, and many others.

ALL FERMENTED BEVERAGES: Beer, wine, champagne, whiskies, rum, brandies, tequila, root beer, ginger ales, as well as all substances which contain alcohol, e.g., extracts, tinctures, cough syrups, and other medications.

ALL CHEESES: Including fermented dairy products, cottage cheese, natural, blended and most pasteurized cheeses, yogurt, buttermilk and sour cream.

ALL MALTED PRODUCTS: Milk drinks which have been malted, cereals and candies which have been malted.

FERMENTS AND MOLDS: Such as soy sauce, truffles, mushrooms.

ANTIBIOTICS: Penicillin and all the synthetic derivatives therefrom, e.g., Ampicillin, Penicillin V&G, Methecillin, Amoxycillin, Carbenicillin, and many other "illins," "Mycin" drugs and related compounds, such as Erythromycin, Streptomycin, Chloramphenicol. Tetracyclines and related derivatives: all the cephalosporin derivatives, Lincocin, and all others derived from molds and mold cultures.

VITAMINS: B, B Complex and multiple vitamins containing B complex. Products containing B_6, B_{12}, irradiated ergosterol (Vitamin D). All products containing Brewer's yeast or derivatives.

2. Substances which contain yeast- or mold-derived additives.

FLOURS which have been enriched. As of January, 1977, the author has been unable to find any national brands free of enrichment. Many states have legislation requiring all flours, pastries, cake mixes, etc., to be enriched if sold for public consumption.

MILK which is enriched or fortified with vitamins.

CEREALS fortified with added vitamins, i.e., thiamin, niacin, riboflavin, etc.

3. Substances which may contain molds as allowed contaminants commercially: fruit juices, canned or frozen. (In preparation the whole fruit is used, some of which may be moldy but not sufficiently to be considered spoiled.) Fresh, home squeezed fruit juices should be yeast-free.

DRIED FRUITS: Prunes, raisins, dates, figs, apricots, etc. Again, some batches may be mold-free, but others will have commercially acceptable amounts of mold on the fruit while drying.

BLACK TEA

DISCUSSION

With the constantly expanding compounding of foods, the addition of "enrichments" or the "fortifying" of others; with the widespread usage of medicaments of diverse nature, but all having a yeast, mold, or fermentation-hydrolysis common denominator; the problem of identification and/or elimination becomes almost staggering. In a vitamin-oriented, alcohol-consuming, antibiotic-swallowing culture, the exposure potential is enormous. The above listings are by no means comprehensive, and the physician and patient must carefully evaluate all unknown or suspect contacts themselves.

The non-enriched cereal grain problem can be approached in at least two ways. In some areas it is possible to obtain flour direct from the mill before the enrichment wafers have been added, if the physician will, by prescription, authorize the procedure. Some "natural foods" type stores carry stone ground, non-enriched

flours which can be purchased in bulk. It is to be hoped
that present laws restricting the sale of non-enriched
flours may be modified to at least permit the sale of such
upon a physician's recommendation.

The information supplied herein is furnished courtesy of D.
Eugene Cowen, M.D., of Englewood Cliffs, Colorado 80110.

Regardless of the exact food an individual is allergic-
addicted to, be it wheat, yeast, or milk, he or she will still
respond to the correct mineral supplement used in our treatment program. If used properly, these minerals will effect a
high level of craving control.

Before I fully understood bread and cheese cravings, a
young man asked me to help him lose weight. He tipped the
scales at just over 500 pounds. His history showed a constant
craving for bread and cheese but not for sweets or other
fattening foods. At first our program was quite successful.
He lost over 150 pounds. Then he gradually started to crave
bread and cheese again. Slowly he lost control of his appetite.
No matter what medication or nutritional supplements we
tried, his weight started to rise again. Psychological support
failed, and eventually he regained his original weight plus
more. Had I known about yeast allergies at that time I could
have easily saved him from this backsliding.

Yeast is everywhere

Yeast is almost impossible to avoid (see box). Yeast is added
to nearly everything; many vitamins contain yeast and, worst
of all, yeast is always in the air.

I once tested a middle-aged woman who complained of
craving bread and cheese. We found her to be allergic to
yeast. At that particular time I was trying to block bread and
yeast cravings by removing all environmental triggers. We
asked her whether her cravings occurred in any particular area
of her house. She said that when she was in her bedroom,

FOODS THAT CONTAIN WHEAT

BEVERAGES: Cocomalt, malted milk, Ovaltine, Postum, and whiskies.

BREADS: Biscuits, crackers, muffins, popovers, pretzels, rolls, and the following kinds of breads: Corn, gluten, graham, pumpernickel, rye, soy, and white bread. *Note:* Rye products are not entirely free of wheat. Whether or not you can use rye will have to be determined on an individual basis if you are found to be sensitive to wheat.

CEREALS: Bran flakes, corn flakes, Cream of Wheat, Crackels, farina, Grapenuts, Krumbles, Muffets, Pep, Pettijohn's Puffed Wheat, Ralston's Wheat Cereal, Rice Krispies, Shredded Wheat, Triscuits, Wheatena, and other malted cereals. Malted cereals are included in the wheat list because for purposes of clinical procedure, barley is considered the same as wheat. There are, however, definite sensitizations to barley malt when allergy to wheat cannot be proved. The reverse is also occasionally true!

FLOURS: Buckwheat flour,* corn flour,* gluten, patent flour, rice flour,* rye flour, white flour, graham flour, lima bean flour,* and whole wheat flour. One should not overlook any mixtures with flour in them!

MISCELLANEOUS: Bouillon cubes, chocolate candy, and all chocolate (except *bitter* cocoa and chocolate), cooked mixed meat dishes, fats used for frying flour-rolled foods, fish rolled in flour, fowl rolled in flour, gravies and griddle cakes, hot cakes, ice cream cones, malt products or foods containing malt, and meat rolled in flour. (*Do not overlook meat fried in fat that has been used to fry meats rolled in flour—particularly in restaurants!*) Also on the list are most cooked sausages (*weiners, bologna, liverwurst, lunch ham, hamburger, etc.*), matzohs, mayonnaise,* pancake mixtures, sauces, synthetic pepper, some yeasts, thickening in ice creams, waffles, wheat cakes, and wheat germ.

PASTRIES AND DESSERTS: Cakes, cookies,* donuts, frozen pies, pies, chocolate candy, candy bars, and puddings.

WHEAT PRODUCTS: Bread and cracker crumbs, dumplings, hamburger mix, macaroni, noodles, rusk, spaghetti, vermicelli, and zwieback.

---

*Read labels carefully. Some of these products contain wheat, others do not.

---

she seemed to get a yen for cheese. I asked her to search for mold in the adjoining bathroom, on the ceilings, and so on, but her search turned up nothing. I didn't see her for several months, until she suddenly appeared in the office one day to tell me she had finally discovered some mold in her bedroom, and that after cleaning it out she lost her desire to nibble cheese—at least while in that part of the house. Apparently rain had run under the windowsill and down the bedroom wall and under the rug near the window. Fungus had grown under the rug and was giving off spores, making the woman susceptible while in its presence.

Yeast in the air

This woman's case illustrates the point that airborne odors and spores can stimulate both hunger and cravings. The smell of bread near a bakery or the odor of cooking starts awakening our senses. Many patients report hunger cravings while preparing dinner. Hunger and cravings are stimulated by the smell even more than the sight of food. This is demonstrated by an old dietician's trick: A patient puts petroleum jelly in both nostrils before cooking dinner, the aromas are blocked, and appetite stimulation is stifled as well.

If you question just how easy it is for the smell of food to get your juices flowing, think how tempting a popcorn stand is, with that fresh buttery aroma wafting through the air. In reality, you don't even have to be *conscious* of an odor for it to trigger a craving. It takes only a few molecules of yeast in your nostrils to create an allergic-craving response. The source of the problem never even reaches the consciousness of the victim. Instead, after being affected by the mold spores, he starts to feel vaguely hungry and thinks it's a spontaneous feeling. If he's really concentrating on an interesting activity, it may take a while for hunger to reach a conscious level, but by then it will have become quite powerful.

Appetites and cravings stimulated by odors can be the result of an allergy to the foods or they can be caused by hypoglycemia (low blood sugar as a reaction to the odors). Increased acid in the stomach can also be stimulated by odors. Rising insulin levels decrease blood sugar, causing hunger and hypermotility of the stomach. Many patients who regularly cook dinner report a churning stomach and a feeling of emptiness at that time, sometimes accompanied by an uneasy burning in the stomach.

IRENE: THE SANDWICH QUEEN

Irene, an early patient of mine, was crazy about sandwiches in a way that resembled Ray Milland's alcoholic binges in the film *Lost Weekend*. Her husband was only vaguely aware of her addiction and admonished her occasionally when he found her gorging on sandwiches. But he witnessed only the tip of the iceberg. Her addiction was extreme, and Irene was cleverly able to keep most of her eating "undercover."

During the day while her husband was gone, she made a number of sandwiches and stashed them throughout the house. A favorite hiding place was in her underwear drawer. Other spots included the laundry room behind the detergents, the back of a bookshelf, or the bottom of a wastebasket. If her husband stumbled onto a stray sandwich, Irene always managed to avoid a confrontation, saying that the sandwich had somehow got "misplaced." She had to hide an extra supply of sandwiches in case some were found, for she didn't dare risk running out. There had to be a backup stock in case her husband or visitors made it inconvenient or awkward to trek to the kitchen. Interestingly, most of her sandwiches contained cheese. Irene, of course, was ashamed of these tactics, and her obsession tormented her, even more because she desperately wanted to lose weight.

She came to our clinic and began a weight control program. During the first interview, however, she avoided all mention of her compulsions. Out of shame and embarrassment she lied to me about her daily intake of carbohydrates.

Many others, of course, suffer from this problem. Some have resorted to induced vomiting to get rid of calories and avoid weight gain. This disease is called bulimia.

After a month on the program, Irene had only lost seven pounds, and then regained it. She bounced up and down. Every time I questioned her about her compliance with the diet, she insisted defensively that she wasn't overeating. In a sense she wasn't. She was taking almost no food at her regular meals so that she could continue with the sandwiches in secrecy.

By the fifth week she could no longer keep up with the deception and finally confessed her sandwich mania. She sincerely believed she had a psychological problem from which no amount of dieting could save her. She asked if I thought she needed psychiatric help.

I explained that the problem wasn't in her mind, it was in her body. Upon testing Irene for food allergies, I discovered she was allergic to yeast. We then gave her the proper supplements, and they managed to counteract the yeast allergy enough so that she could comply with the diet successfully.

ELLIE: THE FRITTERS FREAK

Ellie was a confirmed fritters freak. Apple fritters and bear claws were her downfall, and during times of stress, she could devour them by the boxful. Working as a telephone operator, she sat in the same position all day, and as long as things went well, she could control her cravings. If her supervisor said one cross word, she would leave the building on her coffee break and sneak across the street to the bakery shop. Later, if you happened to call in to her switchboard after such an outing, you might hear a garbled voice with a mouthful of food—Ellie on a fritters binge.

Ellie was obviously out of control. On testing we found her addicted to both sugar (corn) and yeast, so we combined the formulas for sugar craving with the one for bread and cheese cravings and she soon regained partial control. I say partial control because it was especially difficult to gain Ellie's full cooperation. Because of a hormone imbalance, she was always on edge and her emotions were volatile. Her emotions triggered her cravings. If she had a fight with her boyfriend, the end result was a reckless car race to the bakery for a bagful of fresh fritters. The greater the emotional trauma, the greater the fritter fit.

On one occasion, her eating rampage was so intense she began to treat her food as though it were a liquid, swallowing almost without chewing. Some particles caught in her throat, causing a severe choking attack, much the same as what happened to the singer Mama Cass, who succumbed to suffocation. The experience was frightening. Treating Ellie's hormone imbalance was essential before craving control was possible. Later in the book we discuss the effects of hormones on mineral balance.

PAUL: THE BAKERY BUFF

Paul was a young man who suffered from morbid obesity. His condition was so severe that his huge body was all but immobilized by weight in excess of 500 pounds. Paul could scarcely walk, let alone work or function normally; the slightest exertion caused shortness of breath and immediate fatigue. His family accommodated his disability by bringing him food and other necessities while he sat glumly glued to his only link to the outside world—an old television set.

When Paul first came to my attention, I was concerned, for I'd recently heard of a case in which a woman weighed more than 700 pounds—400 of them gained during just one year. The tremendous jump in weight was the result of continual eating, coupled with little physical movement. This person was forced to sleep on two standard-size hospital beds, strapped together, and her upper torso had to remain constantly raised, or breathing became impossible. In spite of this precaution, her respiration became so labored one evening that her parents summoned an ambulance. In spite of valiant efforts by the paramedics to get the woman out the door, her size defeated them. She died as she had lived, trapped in a prison of fat.

When I first saw Paul, I was afraid he was headed for the same fate. His cravings for bakery goods, especially fresh bread and buns, caused him to consume huge quantities of pastry at one sitting, each bite heaped with peanut butter or cream cheese. As you may well imagine, his family was terribly distraught, but they had long since despaired of helping Paul and found it easier simply to give in to his constant demands for more and more food.

But when his health finally deteriorated to the life-threatening point, they brought him to my office in desperation. After some initial counseling with both Paul and his parents, I put him on my program, and for the first time in his life, this helpless—and nearly terminal—patient had his cravings under control and was able to achieve rapid and consistent weight loss.

Paul was so heartened by these results that he began a total fitness program that included exercise and sound nutritional habits. In time, his dedication paid off, and today, Paul is a "free" man, free from a morbidly obese body and the imprisoned life that it dictated. Now, when Paul watches television, it's with a glass of mineral water in his hand and his eye on the clock. For like all normal healthy young men, he has a busy schedule, and not much time for sitting around.

An extra boost

I have often used niacin either separately or together with Min-tran to block bread and cheese cravings. I use 50 mg of niacin every two or four hours. A 50 mg dose seldom causes an uncomfortable rash or itching, and there are usually no other side effects. But if I see a rash, a single aspirin will block the flush in five minutes. If the patients can tolerate the rash and flush, however, I ask them to do so, for the flush has benefits. Some people who are serious buffs of life extension programs intentionally create a niacin flush to give their blood vessels a daily workout. Unfortunately, some doctors not acquainted with the niacin flush have actually sent patients to the hospital in a panic after receiving a call from someone describing such symptoms. Fifty milligrams of niacin is not a high dose, and the flush is both healthful and safe. Ear, nose, and throat physicians often use niacin to assist patients with ear problems, and a few cardiologists have used niacin successfully on patients with high blood pressure. If you don't want to use niacin, you may try the same dose of niacinamide. It doesn't cause a rash, but it is less effective, so you may need a higher dosage. Also keep in mind that the craving could be a combination of sweets craving and bread and cheese cravings, so you may also need some of the items from Chapter 3.

A case of overexposure

What usually sets off yeast cravings is frequent exposure to the addictive items—in other words, pasta, bread and cheese, cookies: anything that starts the cycle, especially if these items are eaten for several meals in a row. Allergies become more intense when there are collections of allergenic foods at different levels of the bowel. Especially if the patient is constipated, there may be six, eight, ten, or more meal residues at different levels along the gastrointestinal tract. You can find more information in Chapter 6.

Emotions also trigger cravings, as most of us are aware. Just how these emotions affect blood chemistry will be discussed later. Hormone changes, too, affect blood sugar, altering the acid-base balance and thus producing cravings; this, too, will be covered in depth later on.

Other allergies

Other allergies, be they to food, to pollen, or to other substances, all may trigger cravings. Diet, medicines, health, weather, and temperature are factors, too. Anything that can start an airborne allergy or contact allergy can start a food craving.

The very best way to stop bread and cheese cravings is to obtain some organic minerals (Standard Process Laboratories) and start with three tablets. You will usually feel an effect within half an hour. Repeat the dose every three hours if the craving has been intense. Keep to this schedule for four days, then you can back off the schedule a bit and use the pills only when you have the cravings. Also, remember to eliminate your exposure to products that contain yeast (see box). If you are faithful in decreasing your exposure to all these foods and the real culprits in particular—cookies, cakes, pasta, Italian foods or Mexican foods containing yeast and wheat —you may find your allergy is less intense and you can rapidly decrease the dosage. You may elect to start the procedure again if and when the cravings return. (Be sure you read the chapters on allergy and yeast because they discuss long-term controls.)

If organic minerals are not available in your local drug or health food store, you may substitute four 7½ grain alfalfa tablets along with an aspirin and a large glass of water. Stick to the schedule described for organic minerals. After four days you will need the pills only occasionally.

When you begin a weight control program, use these products to assist you while you're on the program, because even if you use appetite suppressants, they will have no effect on your cravings.

Obese patients who are trying to lose weight often experience severe attacks of hunger—unrelenting hunger that runs from the time the craver wakes up to the time the individual goes to bed. Some of these patients even awaken in the middle of the night to eat more food. The cause of this behavior appears to be a severe allergic reaction to yeast and/or wheat. Three physiological effects result from this food-allergy reaction.

1. A constant craving for food items that contain yeast or wheat, such as cookies, breads, cheeses, wine, and beer
2. Bloating and water retention (edema)

3. A 50 percent increase in general hunger for all other foods.

Compulsive round-the-clock eating patterns may be broken by taking four organic mineral tablets with one aspirin every three hours for four straight days and avoiding anything containing yeast or wheat during that time.

There is no mystery about why the cravings stop after four days (see Chapter 6 on food allergies). It takes four days for yeast and wheat foods to be completely eliminated from the stomach and intestines. So long as even a small amount of these foods remains in the digestive tract, the cravings will continue. Once every ounce of these two items has cleared the gastrointestinal tract, all cravings disappear. Thus the pills will be needed only occasionally. I can honestly say that I have yet to encounter a failure among patients using this routine properly.

CHAPTER FIVE

How to Stop
Lesser-Known Cravings

While sweets binges steal the limelight, other cravings are just as troublesome to those who suffer from them. Included in this group is the craving for salt, which ranks as the third most common problem, right behind sugar, bread, and cheese. It tends to be more transient in duration and is less intense than the others, so it doesn't rate as much attention.

Other cravings discussed in this chapter include milk and beef, which are equally frustrating to their victims. If we've missed your particular Achilles heel thus far, keep reading, for we don't intend to let even the most remote problems escape attention.

Beef

What could be more surprising than to hear someone complaining about craving beef? Yet I have treated a number of such individuals. Beef is really a rather common allergy because of its protein content. If undigested, as frequently happens, it may become quite allergenic.

Beef and milk are in the same food family; therefore a person who is allergic to milk may also be allergic to beef. Milk allergy is extremely common and so is beef allergy, but the latter is less recognized. Milk, of course, is a product of the female of the species, and veal is also implicated because it represents young beef. Biproducts of beef—gelatin, margarine, and so on—can cause similar allergic reactions.

Although beef cravings are often due to beef allergy, I have discovered that they are also caused by a need for phosphorus. All the patients I've treated have experienced rapid improvement when given products containing phosphorus—in particular, Phosfood liquid, made by Standard Process Labs. Products that have a high phosphorus level include phosphorus liquid and lecithin pearls. Beverages that contain phosphorus, such as diet drinks, do not seem to alleviate the craving.

I instruct my patients to take two 500 to 1000 mg lecithin capsules every three hours, or 20 drops of Phosfood liquid four times a day. Too much phosphorus can cause a calcium deficiency, so balance must be maintained by taking a minimal dose. Phosphorus is also a stimulant, and large amounts can cause nervousness.

Liver has a high phosphorus content and can also be used to block beef cravings. Because most liver comes from beef, one could argue that people would be consuming the very thing they are allergic to. I agree with the logic, but as a practical matter, liver works. I recommend patients take four 3000 mg liver tablets every four hours, and often the cravings disappear after a few days, so treatment can then stop.

Milk

Milk is a fascinating food. It's full of good nutrition but it's also full of sugar and fat, which makes it high in calories. Worst of all, it's highly allergenic. Milk products, such as ice cream and cheese, are also highly allergenic for many people.

One of the most common manifestations of milk allergy is headaches. A number of medical reports have recently appeared concerning milk allergy and migraines.

Sinusitis, which produces a congested "full" feeling in the face and a constant runny nose, is another commonly seen allergic manifestation of milk. Children or adults who are constantly clearing their throats or are frequently sniffing could also be suspected of having a milk allergy. The same is true of diarrhea in children.

There are numerous reasons why one would crave milk. For example, it is reasonable to assume that a calcium-deficient person will seek the calcium contained in dairy products. But we must consider the allergic-addictive possibilities as well.

I don't know whether a craving for milk reflects a deficiency of calcium or an allergic addiction to milk, but we do know that calcium deficiency in animals definitely causes an increased hunger for that mineral. Animals with low parathyroid function also crave foods containing calcium. It seems the drive for calcium can be similar to the properties of other appetite drives.

Doctors in mainland China observed that a low milk intake produced a calcium deficiency in a number of peasants. Pregnant women, especially, showed an affinity for chewing bones from sweet-and-sour dishes. In extreme cases, calcium-deficient patients may even crave chalk or plaster.

In every case I have treated, regardless of the cause, calcium lactate has been the antidote. The patient takes one to four 5 grain (324 mg) calcium lactate tablets every four hours, and the craving disappears magically. I have never had to use anything else for this particular problem, which is good news, for I find milk craving more insidious than others. Milk's reputation as a complete food and a health food is very appealing. Milk is a high-stroking food because it's what Mom used to bring at bedtime or gave you with cookies as a treat. It has fond memories associated with it; milk tastes good and is very satisfying. For all of these reasons and more, it's a very hard food to avoid or give up.

I find milkaholics going back again and again to milk, first because of the psychological reasons mentioned above, and second, because they are still indirectly exposed to it on a constant basis. Almost all bakery goods contain milk, and as we know, any exposure to an allergen will stir up the allergic response. In this case, read the list of foods containing milk (see box) and be aware of how difficult it is to avoid.

FOODS THAT CONTAIN MILK

Baking powder biscuits, baker's breads,[†] Bavarian cream, bisques, blanc mange, boiled salad dressings, bologna, butter, buttermilk, and butter sauces.

Cakes, candies (except hard or homemade), chocolate or cocoa drinks or mixtures, chowders, cookies, cream, creamed foods, cream sauces, cheese of every description,[*] curd, and custards.

Donuts.

Eggs (scrambled) and escalloped dishes.

Foods prepared au gratin, foods fried in batter (*fish, poultry, beef, and pork*), prepared flour mixtures, and fritters.

Gravies.

Hamburgers (homemade), hash, hard sauces, and hot cakes.

Ice creams.

Junket.

Mashed potatoes, malted milk, Ovaltine, Ovomalt, meat loaf, cooked sausages, milk chocolate, and milk, including condensed, dried, evaporated, fresh, goat's, malted milk, and powdered milk.

Omelettes, oleomargarines, pie crust made with milk products, popcorn, popovers, and prepared flour mixtures such as biscuits, cake, cookies, donuts, muffins, pancakes, pie crust, waffles, and puddings.

Rarebits.

"Boiled" salad dressings, sherbets, soda crackers, soufflés, milk or cream soups, Spanish cream, and spumoni.

Whey and waffles.

Zwieback.

When you inquire concerning the presence of milk in any product, put your question in this way: "Do you use butter, oleo margarine, cream cheese of any kind, fresh milk, buttermilk, dried milk, powdered milk, condensed milk, evaporated milk, or yogurt in this food?"

†Not all preparations of these contain milk. You must check this point! *Pareve* breads are milk free.

*Although all cheeses are to be considered as milk products, a patient not sensitive to milk may be found allergic to one or more cheese. Therefore, consider each kind and brand of cheese as a potentially specific allergen.

Ice cream

I usually prescribe three 5 grain (324 mg) calcium lactate tablets here in the same manner as with milk cravings, and the response is gratifying. For example, if patients report going on an ice cream binge every night, I suggest they take three 5 grain calcium lactate tablets after dinner. If they stay up past 11:00 P.M., they probably should take three more tablets at that time.

If the patient can't do without a midnight snack, frozen fruit can hit the spot. If there's a weight problem, the best two fruits are melons and grapefruit. Served chilled, both are tasty and low in calories.

Orange juice

Dr. Theron Randolph, the "father" of food allergy addictions, has probably seen more cases of orange juice allergy than any physician in the world. In Dr. Randolph's recent book, *An Alternative Approach to Allergies*, he describes such a case.

A young teenage boy, prone to temper tantrums and hyperactivity since his first birthday, had been dragged by his parents to a string of child psychiatrists. Interestingly, his siblings, in the same environment, had none of his problems. One psychiatrist said that Tony, being a middle child, didn't get the respect of his older brother or the babying and attention of his younger brother. So, therefore, he was literally crying out for attention.

As time passed, Tony's behavior reached criminal proportions. He frequently lied and stole things, but more alarming, he violently beat the family dog and killed and mutilated another pet. He built model airplanes only to smash them, and apparently enjoyed breaking furniture. One day, while his parents were away, he ripped out a hole in the wall between his bedroom and the living room so he could crawl through. His parents were at their wits' end.

Tony's general history suggested food allergies, and the most important clue in that respect was his tremendous fondness for orange juice. He also craved hard candy. When Dr. Randolph put the boy in the hospital and tested his response to orange juice, his face became flushed. He insulted everyone in sight and demanded to go home. He tried to demolish the hospital room and slapped his mother. In a later test, involving grapefruit, he had a similar but less intense response. He also reacted to peanuts, corn, peas, and bananas. Dr. Randolph ordered him to avoid all of these foods, and, in a short time, there was a dramatic improvement not only in his behavior, but in his schoolwork as well.

Oddly enough, almost no one ever complains of craving orange juice. People usually just say they love it, or that it's an important contribution to a healthy diet. They view it as a health food pure and simple, and never consider its possible toxic effects.

I personally have never seen a case quite so dramatic as Dr. Randolph's, but I do remember one woman I tested who was struck with sudden low back pain several minutes after the test for oranges. She then revealed she'd spent an entire year seeking help for this affliction. She had seen orthopedists, neurologists, and chiropractors—all to no avail. After the test, she eliminated orange juice from her diet, and when

I saw her three months later, she'd had no return of the pain whatsoever.

If you now think that orange juice might not be just a favorite food, but rather a possible allergic addiction, you could use the program in Chapter 3 to stop the cravings. I start my patients on two to four Min-tran tablets every two to four hours depending on the severity of the cravings. Sea kelp tablets can be substituted for Min-tran. To the kelp I add calcium lactate and liver tablets, two to four of each along with the kelp. Occasionally I also add Complex F, two to four tablets along with the above items. Linseed oil capsules can be used in place of Complex F tablets, although they are less effective. Evening primrose oil caps can also be used in place of Complex F capsules.

Be sure to read Chapter 3 for more details. After three days the cravings should be gone, and you should notice remarkable changes. Addictions that reach the intensity experienced by Dr. Randolph's patient probably will require the help of a physician, because individuals like Tony often have multiple allergies, and an unsuspected one could trigger the orange juice reaction all over again.

Marijuana and the "munchies"

One day while under treatment for another ailment, a patient named Jane asked if I knew of anything that would help her with the cravings she got after smoking marijuana—often known as the famous "munchies." I hadn't been asked this question before, so I'd not given it a lot of thought, but I told Jane that marijuana probably depleted the body of a lot of different minerals, and therefore a good mineral tablet might help. She came back the next day to tell me how effective the remedy had been. I don't know exactly what she used, but any good mineral tablet probably would do, if it contains major as well as minor or trace minerals. *Allorganic* from Standard Process Labs is extremely effective. I suggest two to four tablets every two hours until the cravings stop and then one every four hours.

Acid cravings or the desire for something sour

Although the craving for acids is admittedly not a common problem, it's still seen occasionally in some patients, especially those on a diet, and particularly in pregnant women. One theory is that, during pregnancy, the craving for acid foods is due to a need for acetic acid to detoxify the chemical methylguanidine, which is produced by spoiled protein foods. Methylguanidine is a potent alkalizing substance that can cause calcium to leave the tissue fluids. If all that sounds like Greek to you, just note that constipation is a major cause of methylguanidine buildup because decaying foods are retained in the digestive tract. The first step to controlling acid craving is to regulate your system. Urblax from Shockley is effective, and diuretic herb tea like Lace le Beau can be helpful. Bulking agents like bran tablets are also good, and so are stool softeners such as Ducolax. If for some reason none of these is effective, a gentle enema should be tried before using laxatives.

If there's no constipation, try apple cider vinegar; it provides the acetic acid needed by the body and you can take one teaspoon, as needed. You can use 25 mg of riboflavin (Vitamin B$_2$) three times a day because it assists in acetic-acid metabolism. Chlorophyll pearls are also helpful—one could try two capsules every four hours.

Ice

The craving for ice is generally associated with iron deficiency, so the craving should stop when iron is given. But things are not always that simple. A patient of mine, Mrs. R.J., had craved ice for years. In fact, there were very few moments of the day when she didn't have ice in her mouth and a cup of cubes nearby. Every time she came into my office, she brought ice with her, and she admitted that she carried around a cupful even on business and social occasions. My first thought was to prescribe an iron supplement, but

Mrs. R.J. had already tried it on her own, and other doctors had given her iron injections. Although her anemia had temporarily improved, this didn't decrease her desire for ice, and once the iron injections were discontinued, she quickly lapsed back to an anemic condition.

I did some quick checking and found that a deficiency of vitamin B_6 might be a possible cause for her problem. I gave Mrs. R.J. iron injections *and* 100 mg B_6, and after a single day, her desire for ice totally disappeared. As long as she takes B_6, the craving for ice shouldn't return. Once her B_6 reserve is built up, she may go several days without the B_6 with no symptoms, but the craving will gradually well up again. A complicating factor here was a severe hormone imbalance following a hysterectomy, which resulted in the imbalances in iron and B_6.

Another patient whom I treated had pernicious anemia and craved liver as well as ice. I recommend that such patients take 100 mg of B_6 three times a day with their iron tablets. The treatment worked as it had with Mrs. R.J.

Peanut butter

Peanut butter and jelly sandwiches—what kid's lunch pail is without them? There are even songs written praising the joys of this favorite snack. But beware. Commercial peanut butter doesn't consist of just peanuts; it's a composite food with many additives, often including yeast, dextrose, and pure sugar as well as corn oil. This can make it a powerfully addicting substance. If one is addicted to corn sugar and yeast, then peanut butter packs a double whammy. It's not unusual for a peanut butter addict to consume the contents of an entire jar, sometimes on bread, sometimes by the spoonful.

Peanuts are not true nuts. They are a bean from the legume family, and those grown in America often contain extra copper. Peanut butter usually contains a good deal of rancid oil which, combined with copper, creates tremendous amounts of free radicals which are damaging to body tissues. These chemicals age the body rapidly. So, in my opinion, if you want to live long and look young, hold the peanut butter. If that's easier said than done, here's the remedy: The treatment includes the ingredients from Chapter 3 and Chapter 4 combined.

You should reread these chapters for the complete details, but I will make a quick summary here. You might use 5 gr calcium lactate tablets and 150 mcg kelp tablets—four tablets of each every three hours. You may add four tablets of alfalfa and an aspirin.

Other ingredients that may help are 50 or 100 mg tablets of niacinimide and Complex F tablets. We are searching for the ingredients that work in each individual case, and these definitely differ from one patient to another.

Relief should come if doses are taken as recommended. And, of course, keep peanut butter out of your grocery cart; no sense taking chances.

The craving for salt

Since food vendors face cutthroat competition, there are no holds barred when it comes to enhancing taste. And the cheapest way to hook the consumer is by adding salt. The average American gets 10 to 12 grams of salt daily—twice what the body needs. Some eat even more. It's estimated that five grams (½ to 1½ tsp) of salt a day is healthy; more can be harmful. Excessive intake of salt usually starts early in life and continues onward. It may begin before birth if the mother takes in too much salt during pregnancy. Salty baby foods follow, then junk foods during childhood. Adults continue to consume highly flavored pleasure-giving foods and are subjected to a high content of "hidden" salt in prepared foods.

The four types of taste sensors on the tongue—salty, sour, bitter, and sweet—combine to produce taste. Taste is also modified by the smell of the food; this blend of odor and taste is called flavor. Salt affects taste, changing the raw or sour flavors to something more palatable. Additional condiments frequently used for novelty may also contain salt. It's also possible that salt may add something to food that releases the natural odor more easily and thus improves the flavor.

The desire for salt results from pleasure seeking. For example, salty food provides instant gratification, whether it be in the form of potato chips or caviar. Animals, for the most part, will eat for pleasure as well as need, and salt is a universal appeaser.

Additionally, salt is important because the consistency of our blood (and the blood of all mammals) resembles the composition of sea water, though it is less concentrated. Additional salt helps us maintain this balance.

Salt enters our bodies through both liquids and solid food and is excreted through the skin and sweat glands, in saliva, in the stools, and in urine. It is the principal mineral of the body, helping homeostatic mechanisms such as the osmotic pressure of the vascular system and the acid-base balance.

In general, herbivores are more likely to be salt deficient than carnivores, since large areas of the continents are deficient in sodium, and less salt is found in plants than in animals. Many herbivores have demonstrated strong salt affinity, as seen in the popularity of salt licks. Carnivores, on the other hand, are less sensitive to salt since their bodies contain higher levels as a result of eating other animals whose carcasses contain more salt than plants do. Salt appetite, salt hunger, or salt cravings are undeniably real. In the animal kingdom, sodium deficiency is quite common.

Another cause of salt cravings is excessive water intake, and stress also can accentuate such need. Pregnancy and lactation, disease, other mineral imbalances, and dietary changes all put a strain on the body's salt balance.

Symptoms of a salt deficiency are fatigue, lethargy, exhaustion, cramps, low blood pressure, loss of appetite, nausea, constant thirst, and a loss of taste. Some people who have salt deficiencies crave salt, but others don't, and some people don't seem to need it at all.

Salt cravings can be a symptom of a number of unrelated diseases. The underlying mechanism may be unknown, as in the case of sickle cell anemia, diabetes, and various muscle diseases. Because salt cravings often go unrecorded on medical examinations, the prevalence of this phenomenon is not well documented.

Salt depletion will cause salt taste sensors to transmit electrical signals to the brain that may stimulate a search for relief. Stimulating taste buds produce a quest for the salt; this is instinctive rather than learned behavior.

An Australian scientist (Myers, 1967) found that rabbits living in mineral-deficient areas often had strong appetites for wooden pegs soaked in salt.

When we hear people complain of cravings, we immediately think of carbohydrates and sugar, but over the years I have seen a relatively large number of people with salt problems. Some of these people crave both salt and sugar at the same time.

There is some possibility that many individuals with high blood-pressure have a decreased sensitivity to salt and therefore need more salt than the average person in order to taste their food. This decreased sensitivity to salt could be an early sign of impending hypertension.

Here we see the flaw in the innate wisdom of the body. Increased salt intake does *not* restore a true balance to the blood pressure. The low blood pressure in the long run may overcompensate into high blood pressure. If potassium is also taken, the long-term development of high blood pressure can sometimes be avoided. The body is in some respects short-sighted; to achieve balance in the long term, it should increase its desire for potassium—but it doesn't.

Not everyone who eats ample salt suffers as a result; genetics play a strong role. There are, for example, individuals whose intake of salt is high but who have low blood pressure. The cause of occasional salt cravings seems to be adrenal stress—the higher the level of stress, the greater the need for adrenal support. Our adrenals are glands that help us when we are under stress. The stress can be psychological in origin or a result of exposure to pollen or chemicals to which the body is allergic. Physical stress combined with mental stress can demand more support than the adrenal glands can supply, and a need for salt develops. Weakened, overstressed adrenal glands allow the blood sugar and blood pressure to drop, causing fatigue. An increased salt intake could temporarily help the homeostasis in this situation—so we crave salt.

Nutritionists know that salt relates to adrenal glands and that patients with Addison's disease—a disease of poor adrenal gland function—crave salt. They know that stress can cause salt depletion and is accompanied by salt cravings. Another finding is that adrenal cortical hormones, when given, are know to stimulate an appetite for salt.

Richter and Eckert (1938) showed that animals whose adrenal glands had been removed had an increased appetite for salt. When the adrenal gland is depleted, humans are able to detect salt more easily. An underactive adrenal gland, it seems, changes the sensory acuity in most people, and makes them one hundred times better able to detect salt in their diet. These same individuals are one hundred times better able to detect potassium and sugar (sucrose) than people whose adrenal glands are functioning normally.

In patients with an *overactive* adrenal gland (Cushing's syndrome), taste recognition is depressed. There's an inability to obtain normal taste from foods and less of a desire to seek salt.

In a case reported by Wilkens and Richter, a 3½-year-old boy was admitted to the hospital. He ate almost no hospital food and died within a week. An autopsy revealed the cause of death to be adrenal destruction. The boy's history revealed he had been eating huge amounts of salt, literally by the handful. The lack of salt while in the hospital caused death within a week. We know that rats with adrenal insufficiency seek salt solutions and drink from them voraciously.

Richter described, in another paper, a young male patient who would put an eighth-inch of salt on his steaks and add half a glass of salt to his tomato juice. He even made lemonade with salt. Many of Richter's patients did not specifically express a craving for salt but professed to "like" foods that were heavily salted.

When patients of mine report salt cravings, my first thought is to recommend the use of baking soda, since this contains sodium without the chloride, the other half of the table salt molecule. This enables one to avoid a possible rise in blood pressure. It worked well on the first patient I treated, a 45-year-old man. He frequently complained of craving salt, and although it wasn't a constant problem for him, it occurred often enough to cause concern.

When my patient took baking soda tablets from the drugstore, his cravings stopped, and his blood pressure remained stable. He took the baking soda, at my suggestion, only during periods of craving. I tried this remedy on other patients shortly after and it was totally successful.

There may be some concern related to the sodium found in baking soda—does it raise blood pressure? In a report in *Science* (December 9, 1983), two scientists at the University of California, San Francisco, made a study of dietary sodium as a factor in high blood pressure. They found sodium from baking soda caused body swelling (tissue edema) but didn't elevate blood pressure per se. In addition, they found that sodium ascorbate (a form of vitamin C) did not raise blood pressure either. They concluded that chloride in combination with sodium is the culprit in high blood pressure.

Shahied, in *Biochemistry of Foods and Biocatalysts*, says, "Aldosterone from the adrenal gland is affected in pantothenic acid deficiency and there is an increased appetite for salt as the animal cannot adequately retain salt." This condition leads to internal dehydration.

After using baking soda a number of times without encountering problems, I decided to try pantothenic acid, since it is a food for the adrenal glands. I prescribed this substance for a number of patients, and the result was immediate relief from their salt cravings in all cases.

If you get salt cravings occasionally, you may wish to use my technique to stop them. I use 500 mg tablets of pantothenic acid three or four times daily. Sometimes I increase the dosage and shorten the interval if the cravings are severe. Sometimes I use up to 1000 mg of pantothenic acid every four hours. As a backup, keep in mind the use of baking soda.

Two reasons may explain why pantothenic acid plays a role in salt cravings. First, it may act to stimulate the adrenals to increase their output in response to stress, and second, pantothenic acid is used in the production of the hormones released by the adrenal gland. A deficiency of the substance may cause the body's alarm system to overreact. Second, the fact that increased intake of sugars can decrease blood levels of pantothenic acid by 30 percent suggests its ability to metabolize sugar. In other words, if sugar intake is high, pantothenic acid is depleted to metabolize the sugar. Consequently, if the body encounters stress, the pantothenic acid is not there to assist the adrenal gland, and salt cravings may occur.

Cravings for water

The first thought that comes to mind when one hears a complaint of excessive thirst is diabetes mellitus. The physician must rule out diabetes as well as other physical illnesses before assuming that water craving is caused by vitamin or mineral imbalance. One cause of water cravings, especially nocturnal thirst, is salt deficiency. A patient of mine reported she would get up at least two or three times at night to drink water, and when these episodes occurred, she would keep some at her bedside. Occasionally she would have attacks of thirst during the day and would drink four to six glasses of water at a time. On two occasions while traveling by car, she was caught between cities, and there was no water available for over an hour. Her thirst reached panic proportions, and her distress and fears were appropriately severe.

It may be of interest to note that this patient also craved licorice. Europeans used licorice during World War II to treat adrenal cortical insufficiency. It helps one retain both salt and water and is contraindicated in patients with high blood pressure. In this case, the patient appeared to have inadvertently discovered a partial answer to her fluid cravings. However, patients with Addison's disease (poor adrenal gland function), some of whom also complain of thirst, do not report a craving for licorice.

At first I prescribed that this patient take baking soda before she went to bed, and it predictably stopped her thirst and water cravings. Later, when I discovered pantothenic acid deficiency as a cause of salt cravings, I advised her to take 100 mg at bedtime. The results were even more satisfactory.

Pregnancy and cravings

In pregnancy, increased appetite and cravings tend to develop. In *The Hunger for Salt*, Derek Denton (1982) reports a study in which two-thirds of the pregnant women he studied developed specific cravings. The most common obsession was fruit, and sweets ranked second. Also reported were cravings for salty items, as well as for licorice, cheese, and so on. There was also a general increase in thirst, which may have been partially due to increased salt intake.

The level at which there was perception of all four tastes —salty, sweet, sour, and bitter—was higher. This might stem from a zinc deficiency, since aversions to food also develop during pregnancy, and a loss of taste and smell has also been reported by some pregnant women. Decreased taste and smell is often associated with zinc deficiency. Salt cured cravings in a number of cases. Vitamin B_6 in moderate amounts, magnesium, and calcium have also been used successfully to alleviate cravings. Zinc and B_6 seems to be the most effective combination. None of these substances should be taken without the attending doctor's knowledge and permission.

Summing it up

Cravings take away our self-control and put us at the mercy of destructive impulses. As one patient put it, the "monster within takes over." These powerful drives are difficult to understand as well as control. But I find they can all be controlled by being patient and persistent. Craving control is very important to you. Take your time and use different combinations of supplements until you find the prescription that is right for you.

PART THREE

Long-Term Control of Your Cravings

CHAPTER SIX

How Allergies
Can Cause Cravings

Less than a century ago, doctors first began seriously considering the idea that an illness could be related to low resistance to some internal disease. At that point, a new science was born: immunology. In 1905, one physician found cases in which the patient's consumption of common foods contributed to psychological disorders. At the same time, another doctor discovered an allergy to eggs in a young child. Not surprisingly, interest in food-related allergies increased over the years.

The advent of immunology opened the eyes of medical scientists to a disease that was not transmitted from person to person like a virus but was caused by a perfectly natural external substance such as a pollen or food. "Food is good for you," we were all raised to believe. But what is harmless to one body can develop into a toxin in another.

What is a food allergy?

The term *allergy* refers to any altered reaction of the body occurring with time. It is derived from two Greek words meaning "altered reactivity." Today, however, allergists are divided between those who define allergy strictly as a reaction between antigen and antibody and those who support a broader definition. Most of us relate allergy to pollens, dust, molds, and danders. The reactions these substances produce are dramatic and easy to observe and measure in laboratory tests.

Pollens and dust are not so close to us as foods. We humans are more ready to accept an external problem unrelated to our daily lives than we are to accept the idea of an allergy to our favorite pursuit of happiness. Better hay fever than a cheese omelet or a chocolate bar.

What are the symptoms?

Allergists devote most of their attention to respiratory problems. With only 1300 allergists available to treat a population of 250 million Americans, these physicians have their hands full dealing with hay fever and asthma alone. Antihistamines now provide the simplest treatment for inflamed upper respiratory tracts, swollen sinuses, runny noses, itchy eyes, coughing, postnasal drip, or earaches.

Food allergies, however, are far more difficult to diagnose and treat. Their symptoms can sometimes be deceptive and may be mistaken for a pollen allergy. For instance, tearing or reddening of the eyes may be caused by an allergy to eating wheat as well as by an allergy to cat hairs.

Gastrointestinal problems, too, are deceptive. We often blame a stomach ache on last night's pepperoni pizza rather than this morning's glass of milk. An allergy to what is considered the most harmless food can result in diarrhea, constipation, gas, bloating, nausea, vomiting, ulcerative colitis, ileitis, and pain ranging from mild to severe. Food allergies can intensify peptic ulcers and may even mimic gallbladder disease and appendicitis. During an allergy test, a patient of mine became so hysterical after a small dose of wheat that I had to administer oxygen to relieve the symptoms. The same patient reacted so violently to chocolate that she emptied her bladder on her chair. Another patient was so completely incapacitated by chocolate that she was bedridden for twenty-four hours.

We tend to think that chocolate allergy symptoms are confined to a bad complexion, but they can be far more extensive. Chocolate affects more tissues in the body than do inhalants, drug allergies, or infectant allergies.

Food allergies may also be the most common cause of excessive urination, urinary tract infections, prostate disorders, and gynecological problems. Furthermore, such allergies can affect the heart and circulatory system by causing swollen eyelids, irregular heartbeat, and high blood pressure. They even affect the muscle system, causing muscle aches and pains, muscle pain at the nape of the neck, muscle spasms in the lower back, chest pains, abdominal spasms mimicking appendicitis, arthritis and joint pains, swelling, or bursitis.

Last but not least is the neurological allergy, which relates to most of the problems addressed in this book.

Fatigue and sleeplessness are the most common symptoms of food allergy. Often experienced at its worst in the morning, food allergy fatigue can be accompanied by general weakness, drowsiness, and a sensation of heavy limbs often associated with headaches, irritability, depression, and confusion. Such symptoms as moodiness, worrying, poor concentration, indecisiveness, diminished memory, and mental lapses are too frequently confused or combined with hypoglycemia. They can lead to extreme depression, anxiety, and tension, to social withdrawal, to breakdowns, and even to hospitalization.

The most identifiable neurological allergy symptoms are headaches. Everyone knows allergies can cause headaches. But what is less evident is the *source* of allergy. Milk products are one of the worst offenders. You may mistakenly assume that cottage cheese relieves your headache, not knowing that the cream in your coffee may have *started* the headache.

What causes food allergies?

Reaction to food is a more frequent cause of allergic manifestations than is widely accepted. Most Americans at one time or another in their lives are allergic to certain foods. Many allergies start in childhood. You may have inherited your allergy from your family, if other family members show similar symptoms. There have been recorded cases of sensitivity to milk, fruit, vegetables, and fish that reach back two or three generations. One physician discovered egg sensitization in four generations of the same family. The stronger the family history of allergy, the earlier you might experience it. Four basic conditions can be attributed to food allergy: inherited tendencies, exposure, health at the time of exposure, and cross-reactions.

Inherited tendencies. Your susceptibility to food allergy, or your "ability to react," may derive from your parentage. Many times there is a family history to allergy, but the absence of allergies in your family history does not necessarily mean you are immune.

People tend to believe that food allergies occur only among small children or infants, who experience vomiting or stomach aches after eating. Adults don't expect to become allergic and commonly believe that allergies disappear with age. Nothing could be farther from the truth. The older you get, in fact, the more food allergies you are likely to develop, even in the late stages of your life. They are not confined entirely to youth.

Exposure. The more often a person is exposed to a specific kind of food, the more he or she is likely to be prone to allergy. Certain ethnic groups consume heavy doses of bread and milk products. Italians are famous for their pasta, cheese, and breads; Hispanics for their cheese and tortillas. Hence, we find a high incidence of yeast allergy among these groups.

Too much exposure to one kind of food at one time may overwhelm the immune system and trigger the allergic process. The combined assault of chemicals, excessive pollens, dusts, and molds with too much sugar, milk, yeast, or wheat can overload the resistance system to the breaking point.

By and large the most common cause of allergy, other than heredity, is lack of variety in the diet—a widespread problem in U.S. society. Because of our national obsession with speeding up and simplifying food preparation, fast-food chains have rapidly taken over our meal planning. The diet of the average American is becoming more and more repetitious: hamburgers, fries, colas, tacos, candies, and sweets galore, all consumed by a society constantly on the move. These factors lead inevitably to the pathological problems of allergic addiction. Of all environmental exposures, eating the same kinds of food daily over the longest period probably makes the most constant impact. With such eating habits, it is hardly surprising that *anyone* can develop addictive food allergies.

Health at the Time of Exposure. Time after time patients claim their allergies began after a serious health problem or major psychological stress. The immune system is very much affected by stress, and allergy is high on the stress list along with obesity, premenstrual tension, and cancer.

Cross-reactions. Addictive allergies cross-react. A person reactive to potatoes, for instance, may also have difficulty eating tomatoes, green peppers, or eggplant, which are from the same food family. Reactions to foods within the same biological families are common. One food may cause the same reaction as another food in the same family. To name a few allergenic combinations that you might not expect:

asparagus and onions	beef and cheese
coconuts and dates	veal and milk
avocado and cinnamon	eggs and turkey
beets and spinach	butter and gelatin
buckwheat and rhubarb	oysters and snails
yeast and mushrooms	cantaloupe and squash
onions and root beer	pumpkin and watermelon
cabbage and turnips	artichoke and lettuce
broccoli and radishes	safflower oil and tarragon
lentils and licorice	tomatoes and chili
carob and peanuts	potatoes and tobacco
almonds and cherries	oregano and peppermint
alfalfa sprouts and beans	parsley and parsnip
carrots and caraway	cashews and mangos

Any sweets addict may be allergic to raw sugar, cane sugar, or molasses. Similarly, members of another food family that may cause a similar reaction are barley, corn, millet, oatmeal, rice, rye, and wheat.

All these foods tend to cross-react, with no logical relationship that you might expect. Wheat and buckwheat, for example, are *not* in the same family. If you are wheat allergic, you can eat all the buckwheat you want without precipitating any reaction. Milk allergy can also elicit some reaction from beef, veal, buffalo, goat, lamb, or mutton.

Food addiction

One hidden symptom strongly differentiates food allergies from other allergies—food allergies can be *addictive*. Like the cocaine addict who snorts continuously to temporarily avoid withdrawal symptoms, foodaholics consume an addictive food on repeated occasions for the same reason. They are on a continuous "maintenance dose," subconsciously acting to keep themselves symptom free. A person whose poison is milk will have milk for breakfast on cereal, yogurt for lunch, and some form of cheese at dinner. By frequently eating the addictive substance, the individual can maintain an "up" feeling for a very long time. The only difference between a food addiction and a drug addiction is the degree of severity. All people are susceptible to addictions if the intake of certain substances continues in large enough doses for a sufficient length of time.

Paradoxically, some foodaholics may never consciously *crave* any particular food. They have merely arranged their eating habits so that the unrecognized addictive food is always included in their meals.

Food addicts seldom if ever seek professional help. They are oblivious to the cause of their problems and seldom suspect they *have* a problem. Like the classic alcoholic, foodaholics possess a talent for self-deception, ignoring the degree and extent of their problem. Unlike the drug addict who can clearly identify his or her addiction, the food addict may be hooked on a number of foods and without recognizing the fact.

Categorically, the worst food addictions are to food and drug combinations such as cigarettes, alcohol, coffee, and chocolate. Pure foods, particularly sugars, are a close second.

Then come starches, proteins, and oils, which are the least addicting. Whatever your poison, it is always a "feel-good food." It is your favorite, the most appealing, and the one you're most likely to abuse that hooks you.

Some experts who support the concept of food-allergy addiction estimate that up to nine out of ten Americans have some form of food allergy. I would make a more conservative estimate, but certainly over 50 percent. The addiction can grow stronger with time, and old addictions can stimulate new ones.

Food allergies can cause nervousness, an indirect link to overeating. Hyperactive children often crave food and drink. One telltale sign is waking up in the middle of the night and feeling compelled to eat before going back to sleep.

How long does a food allergy reaction last?

Depending on the interaction between allergens, symptoms can continue from seven to ten days, sometimes longer, as is often seen with wheat. It takes four days for food to pass through the gastrointestinal tract—longer if the patient does not have a normal pattern of bowel movements.

If you are frequently exposed to the same food, you may carry four or five doses spaced at different intervals along the gastrointestinal tract, thus further prolonging the reaction. Symptoms from a single intake of food can continue for a few hours or, more likely, from one to seven days. For example, hives can develop three hours after eating loganberries but, as I have seen in one patient, they can last for an entire week.

Obesity and cravings

Obese individuals tend to view their so-called nervous eating habit as psychological in nature. It never occurs to them that their cravings are based on a *physiological* need to stop withdrawal symptoms. Nor do they suspect their nightly binges may be a response to withdrawal symptoms that develop when the high from dinner wears off.

Some individuals wake up in the middle of the night after withdrawal pains become so intense they can't sleep. Only the needed "right" food can get them back to sleep again. Many overweight people suffer from a fluid retention (edema) problem due to food allergy.

Let's consider a hypothetical quarrel at the dinner table. Your angry outburst at your mate could have been caused by a neurological reaction to a food you are eating. In turn, your irritation could cause overeating. The more your emotions rise, the more you eat in frustration.

On the opposite side of the coin, there are those people who become nervous from certain foods and overeat to calm themselves. We are all familiar with "nervous eating," but surprisingly, some foods cause the very nervousness that leads to the overeating. If you don't suspect the food as the cause, it will not occur to you to avoid the offending item. So you remain perpetually nervous, overeating and overeating to escape the nervousness brought on by the allergenic food—a vicious cycle. It's no wonder people get fat.

Many people eat when they get tired. I have seen many patients compelled to overeat because they "need the energy." They are chronically tired and look for anything that might give them a lift. When I discover which food allergens caused the fatigue, I simply remove that food from their diet. Their energy returns, and the weight problem is easier to control.

Allergists can turn cravings on and off. They employ a method that provokes an allergic reaction in the patient by using extracts of the food to which he or she is allergic. Then they remove the cravings by using neutralizing doses of the same extract. Once I treated 34 patients for sugar and chocolate cravings. When placed on an allergy desensitization program, nearly every patient reported loss of cravings. A year later, I contacted a few who reported they still had no recurring desire for sugar or chocolate. Desensitization treatments are not the only approach to cravings, but they are certainly effective.

One very important phenomenon I have witnessed in numerous cases: *When a specific craving exists, the overall hunger level increases as well.*

How to determine if you have a food allergy

Do you see yourself in any of the following situations?

1. You feel uncomfortable if you miss or are late for a meal, especially late in the day or into the evening. When you do eat, you "feel good." You usually include some favorite food in the meal, such as bread, cheese, or a dessert. You don't feel complete without them. You may binge at times.

2. You always keep a commonly eaten item stashed at home. If you're out of some coveted sweets on a stormy night, you'll drive through rain and thunder to get them. You are afraid to run out or be without. You may need that treasured item close at hand for emergency snacks.

3. Your cravings are so strong you feel you could never live without a particular food. You find it impossible to stick to a diet. You call yourself a junk-food junkie.

If you can honestly answer "yes" to most of any one paragraph above, you may need to seek professional help. If you visit an orthodox allergist, you will probably not find a favorable reception to the idea of food allergy-addictions. The allergist will probably conduct skin tests, which will work well for pollen and dust but reveal nothing about possible food allergies. Cytotoxic tests are rarely performed with enough competency to be accurate.

If you visit a clinical ecologist, he may use provocative tests to observe reactions to small samples of ingested food. A drop of a suspected allergen is placed under the tongue to determine whether you respond with symptoms the food might be producing during daily intake at home or office. If wheat causes a reaction in the bronchi, then sublingual wheat may cause coughing or wheezing during the test. Any provoked reactions can be neutralized immediately before testing is resumed. There are a few clinical ecology units around the United States that provide such tests, usually associated with a hospital. In the case of more severe allergies, patients can be admitted to the hospital unit for more complete testing.

A do-it-yourself-at-home test

CAUTION: *If you have severe health problems such as asthma, diabetes, epilepsy, or depression, you should not risk taking this test.*

First try a total fast for three days using only spring water (no juices). You can do this if you're hearty. If you get too many withdrawal symptoms, take an Alka-Seltzer, some baking soda, or the other items at the end of this section.

If you are not able to fast, then keep to a simple diet of unrefined carbohydrates, protein, and vegetables. Do not eat the foods you will be testing yourself for. Read labels and avoid any traces of these foods in other products. If you don't take serious precautions, the test will be indecisive and a waste of effort. Avoid caffeine. One way to stave off a coffee fix is to take baking soda tablets, one every hour for four days. You can obtain these at any pharmacy.

Your body must be completely free of your addictive foods. Unfortunately, wheat can remain in the bowels for up to two weeks. Take laxatives during your dieting or fasting period. For the right test results, the bowels *must* have no trace of the addictive foods.

Now you are ready to begin your allergy test:

1. Make a list of the foods you want to test.

2. Buy your foods from a health food store, if you can, to avoid insecticides, herbicides, coloring agents, preservatives, and waxes which may also cause allergic reactions and confuse the results. Use fresh, frozen, or bottled food but no cans, as they give off metals to which you may react. Be sure there are no added ingredients, particularly sugar. Plastic-wraps foods, which may absorb chemicals from the wrap, should also be avoided.

3. Take care in preparing foods. Ocean food such as shrimp or fish should be broiled, baked, roasted, or steamed. Eggs should be boiled or poached. Eat vegetables and fruits raw.

Juices should be freshly squeezed. Don't add pepper, catsup, mustard, sugar, honey, spices, vinegar, or anything else to what you eat or drink. Nuts should be unprocessed. Boil cereals; you can test wheat or oatmeal as a cereal, but avoid yeast. Boil barley in spring water to test malt. To test sugar, dissolve two tablespoons of it in a glass of spring water; for chocolate, eat only unsweetened "baking" chocolate, or grate two to three one-ounce squares into a glass of ice-cold spring water. To test yeast, use baker's yeast or brewer's yeast in cold spring water.

4. Test foods every two hours. The tested portion should be four times the customary size for average meals. Drink only spring water, no beverages. Salt is permissible. Touch no other food. Test each suspicious item by eating enough in one twenty-minute sitting to fill you up.

5. Observe your reactions and write down the symptoms, noting the time you tested the food and how soon the reactions occurred. If you read a book or magazine, you may notice blurred vision. You may experience symptoms in the first twenty minutes, but symptoms usually start within the first hour. Most will occur within four hours after eating. After the test, review your records. If your reactions were severe you will probably need more testing for chemicals, molds, and other substances, so make arrangements with a doctor. If you don't wish to test yourself but you want help, see the last chapter for ways of reaching recommended professionals.

6. Prepare a neutralizer by mixing two parts Arm & Hammer Baking Soda with one part potassium bicarbonate, which is available from your pharmacist.

7. Allow the reactions to run their course and keep a record.

If you have a serious addictive allergy, your withdrawal symptoms may become very uncomfortable. Consult your physician if your reactions become too extreme. Meanwhile, take two tablespoons of baking soda mixture (item 6) in 16 ounces of water and drink immediately. This will neutralize the reaction. Don't test a food for one hour after taking baking soda. Taking two Alka Seltzer Gold tablets in a glass of water also works well. Don't take any alkaline salts if you have a heart or kidney condition. Another excellent way to neutralize food allergy symptoms is to take one teaspoon of vitamin C crystals dissolved in a large glass of water. It usually eliminates symptoms in five to ten minutes.

How do I know which foods to check for?

You should check all high-calorie foods and those you eat most often or are most exposed to, such as corn or wheat. Any favorite food that you eat more frequently than once every three days should be put on your "suspicious food" list, even though you may think you have no real difficulty

---

A TYPICAL ALLERGY TESTING SCHEDULE

Day One: Have coffee first if desired, six boiled or poached eggs for breakfast, two baked potatoes for lunch, and 12 ounces of tuna for supper. Three hours after supper, eat three shredded wheat rolls.

Day Two: Three glasses of milk for breakfast, cottage cheese and an assortment of other cheeses for lunch, beef for supper. Three hours after dinner, have two oranges.

Day Three: Chocolate for breakfast, organic peanut butter for lunch, chicken for dinner. Three hours after dinner eat two cubes of baker's yeast.

Day Four: Oats for breakfast, four tomatoes for lunch, pork for dinner. Three hours after dinner fresh or dried soybeans. (Soybean products are the number one cause of allergies in people who eat "health foods.")

Day Five: Three tablespoons cane sugar in spring water for breakfast, corn for lunch, shellfish for supper. Three hours after supper, eat lettuce.

with that food. And naturally, don't forget to check the foods you crave or are the most hungry for.

The following are the most common foods that cause allergic reactions:

apples	chocolate	peanuts
beef	eggs	pork
cane sugar	green beans	potatoes
carrots	lettuce	soy products
chicken	milk	tomatoes
coffee	oats	wheat
corn	oranges	yeast

Avoid these foods for at least five days before the test so that your body is free of residual effects and your test reactions will be reliable. A typical testing schedule is shown in the box.

Any foods that produce no allergic responses in you during this time can be used freely during the rest of the test. They can be eaten with the foods you are testing. Any foods you find that produce positive symptoms should be excluded for the rest of the test.

What kind of symptoms should I look for?

General symptoms you should watch out for include the following. All demonstrate a definite neurological allergy.

Overactivity: You feel nervous, irritable, or aroused.
Underactivity: You feel sedate, quiet, bored, tired, or sleepy.
Hunger: You develop an increased appetite.
Personality changes: You experience a change in your behavior, such as increased anger or fear.

Your symptoms can be divided into two categories: "subjective symptoms," or nonvisible sensations; and "objective symptoms," or visible sensations. Table 1 shows the symptom list used in my clinic.

Table 1

SUBJECTIVE AND OBJECTIVE SYMPTOMS OF ALLERGY

Subjective Symptoms	Objective Symptoms
Nausea	Hiccups
Headache	Wheezing
Flatulence (gas)	Coughing
Itching	Sweating
Numbness	Herpes ("cold sores")
Unsteady on feet	Burping
Dizziness	Flatulence ("gas")
Fatigue	Change in skin color
Pain in parts of body	Rashes
Dry mouth	Hives
Thirst	Crying
Disturbance of smell	Rubbing eyes
Blurring of vision	Runny nose
Spots before eyes	Circles under eyes
Metallic taste	Lines under eyes
Itching of eyes	Vagueness
Itching of mouth or throat	Faraway look
Ringing of ears	Fast heartbeat
Bloating	Irritability
Joint pains	Flushing
Pressure on chest	Eczema
Difficult breathing	Tenseness
Swelling of mouth or throat	Paralysis
Nose open or closed	Circulatory collapse
Irritability	Swelling
Chilliness	Stuffiness
Depression	Sinusitis
Increased appetite	
Mental confusion	
Mental alertness	

Some subtle changes to look for:

Of all the symptoms listed above, those of a psychological nature are the most difficult to discern. Take, for example, the case of a clinic patient who was tested for her addiction to chocolate. A test dose of a chocolate solution was applied under her tongue in varying concentrations. The ensuing results were reported:

1st dose: The patient complained of sudden hunger.

2nd dose: The same hunger continued for about ten minutes, then suddenly disappeared.

3rd dose: There was no reaction. This turned out to be the neutralizing dose.

4th dose: The chocolate tasted a bit flat and the patient reacted with a flash of anger, objecting strenuously to the way the test was being given. Though she seemed in control, her face betrayed her irritation.

5th dose: The patient became even more incensed, this time totally losing control.

6th dose: The anger disappeared.

At this point the nurse repeated the same dosage, and the patient complained of splitting headache. Then the nurse readministered the *third* (neutralizing) dose—the headache quickly disappeared.

You can see the subtle relationship of food to personality changes. If you flare up at your husband or wife during dinner, the problem may not be what he or she has said but what you ate—brought on by a food allergy. When you take this do-it-yourself allergy test, be very aware of subtle changes.

The next step

Now that you have identified your food allergies, what can you do about them?

First, decide whether they are mild or intense. If your

cravings are very frequent or constant, you probably need help from a knowledgeable physician. If you suffer from permanently fixed food allergies, these too will require professional attention. An allergist can prescribe a dose of cromolyn sodium to help control symptoms of food allergy or cravings. Neutralizing treatments can be administered in the same way pollen allergies are treated.

If self-help is appropriate, the three ingredients I have found to bring quick relief are calcium lactate, kelp, and alfalfa. Review Chapters 2 and 3 for ways to use these materials. Two to four tablets of each taken when the cravings start is very useful, but when you reread Chapters 3 and 4 you may also want to add Complex F, niacinamide, or other additional supplements to augment the above items. Now that you know how each food affects you, you can readily block symptoms such as headaches.

In addition to those methods reviewed, you may use vitamin C (sodium ascorbate) in powdered form to block the cravings. Taking 4000 mg (one teaspoonful) in a large glass of water at the first sign of a craving works quite successfully for many patients. The dosage must be adjusted to each patient's needs. Some side effects may limit the use of vitamin C for some people. It may cause an upset stomach, cramping if the body is low in potassium or calcium, or sometimes water retention. Regardless, vitamin C remains a powerful control device for cravings.

Long-term controls

Decreasing your overreactivity to allergenic foods demands a regimen of long-term abstinence. The longer you can manage to avoid them, the more your body will acquire a higher tolerance for them, depending on the intensity of your cravings. On the average, three months will be enough for milder cravings, up to one year for stronger ones. After that, try not to indulge yourself more than twice in one week. *Use the techniques given in this book to block any return of cravings during this abstinence period.*

If you are just coming off a diet, you may find you have been off the offending foods long enough to have built up a tolerance for the addicting foods. You won't have much trouble keeping your weight down for a few months. But with the passing of time, you may become more careless. You may begin to eat the addicting foods more often. By doing so, you reestablish the body's hyperreactivity, and the allergy addictive cycle starts all over again. My advice when you finish a diet is to exercise caution. Do not reintroduce allergenic foods into your diet more than once every four days.

Chocolate is fairly easy to control in this manner, with one exception. Women who have premenstrual tension can be triggered back into chocolate cravings by the hormone imbalance. This leaves them several possibilities. They can either seek help from a professional or consult one of the many books (including this one) that describe nutritional supplements that can block premenstrual symptoms.

In the case of a more common craving for corn syrup, you should make a conscientious effort to avoid all refined sugar as well as corn sugar, alcohol, corn, popcorn, and so on for 90 days. Beyond that, they should be used *sparingly* for six months to one year.

Granted, breaking the sugar habit is difficult. Avoiding bread, cheese, yeast, wheat, and milk is much harder. It is nearly impossible to avoid all combinations of these substances. The best course of action is to reduce your intake to the minimum for 90 days and take 4000 mg of vitamin C and 100 mg of vitamin B_6 three times a day to counteract your compulsion to eat anything containing yeast (especially), wheat, or milk.

The most difficult allergy of all to treat is *yeast*. Avoidance requires effort sometimes beyond human patience. To deal with yeast cravings, consult Chapter 8.

Keep one thought in mind: You have to give to get. The more effort you put into this program, the more free you will be of your allergy cravings.

To help you avoid allergic food combinations, the following checklist in the box will serve as a guideline to animal and plant foods in the same family.

FOOD FAMILIES: ANIMAL AND PLANT

ANIMAL FOODS

Mollusks

Abalone
Clam
Mussel
Oyster
Scallop

Crustaceans

Crab
Crayfish
Lobster
Shrimp
Squid

Amphibians

Frog

Fish

Anchovy
Barracuda
Bass
Bluefish
Buffalo
Bullhead
Butterfish
Carp
Catfish
Caviar
Chub
Codfish
Croaker
Cusk
Drum
Eel

Flounder
Haddock
Hake
Halibut
Harvestfish
Herring
Mackerel
Mullet
Muskellunge
Perch
Pickerel
Pike
Pollack
Pompano
Porgy
Rosefish
Salmon
Sardine
Scrod
Scup
Shad
Shark
Smelt
Snapper
Sole
Sturgeon
Sucker
Sunfish
Swordfish
Trout
Tuna
Weakfish
Whitefish

Reptiles

Turtle
Snake

Mammals

Beef
  Butter
  Cheese
  Cow's milk
  Gelatin
  Veal
Goat
  Cheese
  Goat's milk
Mutton
  Lamb
Horsemeat
Rabbit
Squirrel
Venison

Birds

Chicken
  Chicken eggs
Duck
  Duck eggs
Goose
  Goose eggs
Grouse
Guinea hen
Partridge
Pheasant
Squab
Turkey

PLANT FOODS

Grains

Barley
  Malt
Cane
  Cane sugar
  Molasses
Corn
Corn oil
Corn sugar
Corn syrup
Cornstarch
Dextrose
  (Glucose)
Popcorn
Oats
Rice
Rye
Sorghum
Wild rice
Wheat
  Bran
  Gluten flour
  Graham flour
  Wheat germ

Spurge Family

Tapioca

Arrowroot Family

Arrowroot

Arum Family

Taro
  Poi

Composite Family

Artichoke
Chicory
Dandelion
Endive
Escarole
Head lettuce
Leaf lettuce
Oyster plant

Legumes

Black-eyed pea
Kidney bean
Lentil
Lima bean
Navy bean
Pea
Peanut
  Peanut oil
Soybean
  Soybean oil
String (green)
bean
Wax bean

Acadia
Licorice
Senna

Mustard Family

Broccoli
Brussels sprouts
Cabbage
Cauliflower
Celery cabbage
Collard
Horseradish

Kale
Kohlrabi
Mustard
Radish
Rutabaga
Turnip
Watercress

Gourd Family

Cantaloupe
Casaba
Cucumber
Honeydew
Muskmelon
Persian melon
Pumpkin
Squash
Watermelon

Lily Family

Aloes
Asparagus
Chive
Garlic
Leek
Onion

Goosefoot Family

Beet
  Beet Sugar
Spinach
Swiss Chard

Buckwheat Family

Buckwheat
Rhubarb

Potato Family

Chili
Eggplant
Green pepper
Potato
Red pepper
  Cayenne
Tomato

Morning Glory Family

Sweet potato
Yam

Sunflower Family

Jerusalem
  artichoke
Sunflower seeds
Sunflower oil

Pomegranate Family

Pomegranate

Ebony Family

Persimmon

Rose Family

Blackberry
Dewberry
Loganberry
Raspberry
Strawberry
Youngberry

Mint Family

Marjoram
Mint
Peppermint
Sage
Savory
Spearmint
Thyme

Pepper Family

Black pepper

Nutmeg Family

Nutmeg

Ginger Family

Cardamom
Ginger
Turmeric

Pine Family

Juniper berries
Pine nuts

Orchid Family

Vanilla

Parsley Family

Anise
Caraway
Carrot
Celeriac
Celery
Coriander
Dill
Fennel
Parsley
Parsnip

Birch Family

Filbert (Hazelnut)
Oil of birch
  (Wintergreen)

Mulberry Family

Breadfruit
Fig
Hop
Mulberry

Maple Family

Maple sugar
  Maple syrup

Palm Family

Coconut
Date
Sago

Lecythis Family

Brazil nut

Poppy Family

Poppy seed

Banana Family

Banana

Apple Family

Apple
  Apple pectin
  Cider vinegar
Pear
Quince
  Quince seed

Plum Family

Almond
Apricot
Cherry
Nectarine
Peach
Plum
  Prune

Grape Family

Grape
  Cream of tartar
  Raisin

Madder Family

Coffee

Tea Family

Tea

Pedalium Family

Sesame oil
Sesame seeds

Myrtle Family

Allspice
Cloves
Guava
Paprika
Pimiento

Mallow Family

Cottonseed
Okra (gumbo)

Stercula Family

Cocoa
  Chocolate

Walnut Family

Black walnut
English walnut
Butternut
Hickory nut
Pecan

Cashew Family

Cashew
Mango
Pistachio

Beech Family

Chestnut

Fungi

Mushroom
Yeast

Miscellaneous

Honey

Source: Data from Dickey, Lawrence D., ed., *Clinical Ecology* (Springfield, Ill.: Charles C. Thomas, 1976). Courtesy of Charles C. Thomas, Publisher. As adapted in *Coping with Your Allergies*, by Natalie Golos and Frances Golos Golbitz with Frances Spatz Leighton (New York: Simon and Schuster, 1979). By permission of Simon and Schuster.

CHAPTER SEVEN

How Fungus
Can Cause Cravings

For our purposes, the terms "yeast," "mold," and "fungus" can be used interchangeably. Yeasts are considered plants but have some characteristics of animals. Some scientists see them as a combination of both.

Yeast: The "man-eating" plant

It's easy to think of people ingesting plants; it is less easy to imagine how a plant could eat someone, and yet that is essentially what yeasts do.

The species of mold called *candida albicans* has no roots through which it can receive water and the other nutrients, but it does contain enzymes that are capable of digesting material from the human body. Mold is probably the most tenacious survivor in the universe. It's found everywhere in nature, even in the soil. It grows on nearly all surfaces that contain any kind of organic material. To reproduce, yeasts release enormous amounts of small particles called spores, which float through the air, when the atmospheric temperature and humidity provide favorable conditions.

Since these molds grow on anything that has been alive, they will grow on the surface of all animals, including humans. They also grow, as you know, inside animals and humans. Different families of yeasts infect humans, and in a single person there can be four, five, or more strains of fungus at one time, although each part of our body seems to attract only one type. The gastrointestinal tract may play host to one kind of mold called *Candida*, our tonsils and our respiratory tract to another variety called *Aspergillus*, and our feet to another fungus called *Trichophyton*. Women know *Candida albicans* under the name of *Monilia*, because that's the most common type found in vaginal infections. Parents may know it under the name of *thrush*, which is a fungus of the mouth commonly found in children. These plants have been growing in us with great success, but until now they have not been thought to cause severe health problems. The disease of being infected with this mold is called *candidiasis*.

The whiz kid of the vegetable world

Candida lives inside the large intestine of nearly all of us. It is quite canny. Although it is a "plant," it behaves almost like an animal: It uses oxygen like an animal, has an animal-like nucleus in each cell, and has a similar metabolism.

King of the plants
vs. king of the animals

For more than ten thousand years, we humans have been toying and experimenting with yeast. We started by using it for fermentation and baking. Then we decided that we could domesticate these plants and use them like farm animals to assist our food chain. We began to use yeast for the consumption of grain on a regular basis, that is, in breads. There had always been large amounts of these molds in the air around us, but now we began to put them inside our bodies, in huge doses.

Man has made serious mistakes throughout history. One of his biggest may have begun only recently when he began to use large amounts of antibiotics. With the onset of their use, both directly and indirectly (such as through food—beef, poultry, eggs, fish, and milk), man opened up Pandora's box, and the yeast went crazy. They began to feast on us like characters in a horror movie. And now we have literally become sick of them.

Man versus yeast

In the past, man had established a stand-off with the yeasts. They were present on his skin and on his mucous membranes (such as in the intestine and the respiratory tract), but he had been able to control them. Occasionally he might lose control. The fungus would dash into his bloodstream and spread throughout the body, and this caused serious problems. But for the most part, man and *Monilia* have been able to coexist.

A delicate balance

The yeasts are usually willing and able to take advantage of any form of weakness. Any disease that weakens the immune system makes it susceptible to yeast growth. Common examples are cancer and AIDS. It you have a disease that stresses the immune system, and then you additionally attack the disease with immunosuppressant drugs, the body has no defenses left against the yeasts, and they start taking over. They further weaken the individual and contribute to his ultimate death.

How does an unwanted fungus get "on board"?

When the spores of fungi such as *Candida* travel through the air or through some other contact source, they invade our nose or mouth and attempt to colonize on our mucous membranes. The body responds by rejecting the invader—for example, by coughing or sneezing.

First of all, the body uses mucosal immunity, which means

that materials produced by the cells of the mucous membranes fight off the invader. In healthy individuals, the mucous membranes have a coating of mucous and immunoglobulin that helps battle the fungus. In addition, most persons have antibodies against this type of yeast.

Unfortunately for most of us, this struggle usually ends in a stand-off, in that the yeast does get a beachhead, but is not able to proceed inland. Man, on the other hand, is able to keep the yeast from invading further but doesn't have the capacity to destroy it completely with his present immune system. Cultured samples of saliva from almost all humans show the presence of small colonies of *Candida*, even though they are not attacking the body in full force. Occasionally an area will simply give in; the yeast will spread wildly. An example of this would be a case of vaginitis.

It has been found that the key ingredient in the success of this yeast landing on and staying on our bodies is its ability to adhere to the mucous surface. But then it must also compete with other microorganisms, such as bacteria, for the food supply available.

Antibiotics: A mixed blessing

It's an easy job, however, for the yeast to attack a person who has a poor immune system. When a person becomes unhealthy for any reason, such as illness or stress, he is open to a successful invasion by the yeast. But what really helps *Candida* and its relatives grow is antibiotics. If we take an antibiotic and kill off the yeast's competitors (antibiotics kill only bacteria, not yeast), then *Candida* is given a green light.

The sea of spores

We are living in a sea of fungus spores. And this troublemaker appears to stay with every one of us from birth until death. We have been living in this sea of spores since our species began. We know that it was a problem even centuries ago, because the ancient Greeks wrote of both oral and vaginal infections, and although they did not diagnose the problems as such, they did describe the exact symptoms that we see in patients today.

Many people live their entire lives with mold growing in their bodies, with no apparent ill effects. Luckily, they have an unusually strong immunity to the mold. For many others, however, the yeasts easily establish an infection. Oftentimes it occurs on the skin, or under the nails of the fingers or toes. When entire colonies begin to grow, we have athlete's foot or other diseases. Many times they are only a nuisance, but anyone who has suffered from these infections knows how very difficult they are to eradicate.

Waves of toxins

These symptoms are mild in comparison to what can happen when the *products of this fungus* get into our blood. When its products get past our mucous membranes and into the body, they begin to act allergenically and to affect other organs. Some scientists call this an allergic response, and others call it a toxic response to the invasion.

Other organs, far from the original site, can be affected as well. Each organ of the body has a different degree of susceptibility, but the weakest systems are the ones most often affected in the earlier stages.

AN "OLD" DISEASE REDISCOVERED

Norma was a 29-year-old woman afflicted with dizzy spells. She'd been to various doctors, and tried a number of treatments for an inner ear disease (labyrinthitis) but without success. A friend told her that doctors who practice clinical ecology take a different approach to such symptoms, so she decided to give one a try.

The doctor she chose took a detailed history and ordered a number of tests. When the results were in, he prescribed a dietary change and some medication. Within ten days the dizziness had totally disappeared. In addition, something unexpected occurred. For years, Norma had been suffering from sugar and chocolate cravings. As a result her weight had risen from a trim teenage level of 115 pounds to a matronly 160 pounds. She had reduced her weight several times but never permanently. She always regained the weight within a year or two because of her obsession for sweets. After treatment for her ear infection, Norma noticed that she no longer craved sugar and chocolate, and her weight control was greatly improved.

During one of her visits to the doctor's office, Norma was sitting in the waiting room, chatting with another patient. Agnes was fifty-four. Her original problem had been fatigue, and it was getting progressively worse. She had visited a number of health food stores and had been put on the customary megavitamin regimen. She'd also visited several doctors. One had given her a stimulant. Another had given her a thorough examination, complete with lab tests, but found nothing and had merely advised her to try to get more rest, and perhaps take up a hobby to relieve stress.

Agnes, too, had been referred to the clinical ecologist by a friend who had been helped by this medical discipline. Both of these women were found to have a fungus infection in the gastrointestinal tract. The fungus involved was *Candida albicans*.

As Norma and Agnes talked, they compared notes on the changes in their hunger patterns along with the improvement in their symptoms. They were surprised that one disease could be responsible for such a variety of symptoms, and they also noticed that their cravings had totally disappeared when their health improved. It's not uncommon for a patient to suffer multiple symptoms, only one of which is major. And when the major symptom is treated successfully, a number of minor symptoms may disappear as well. For example, a patient with high blood pressure may also complain of fatigue. When the blood pressure comes down, the fatigue often disappears. The patient naturally believes that the fatigue is related to the high blood pressure, but it may in fact have been caused by something else.

Infections as a cause of cravings

Changes in appetite caused by disease may seem a bit far-fetched. In fact, though, it's becoming more common to find patients who are allergic to a number of environmental chemicals and who also have excessive appetites and cravings.

A number of doctors who treat candidiasis successfully have reported that some of their patients are having fewer weight problems, less water retention, and an absence of cravings, when candidiasis is cleared up. These doctors are not purposely treating patients for weight control, so they merely consider it an interesting aside. However, for the bariatrician, the doctor who specializes in weight control, this observation can be important.

It should be pointed out that not all cravings for sugar or chocolate are *Candida* associated. However, it's my experience that many of the cravings that we now see are related either directly or indirectly to the *Candida* phenomenon (see box).

Some clinical ecologists, while treating candidiasis, have observed that one of the major signs of improvement is a decrease in the patient's sugar cravings. Clinical ecologists, however, are more concerned with other symptoms and are often not concerned with the cravings. But more and more doctors are using the lessening of craving as an indication that the disease is being treated successfully.

Patients only slightly affected by candidiasis may have only one symptom: unexplainable cravings. This information should be of interest to people who suffer cravings in addition to excessive hunger. It's not just the cravings that become a problem, it's the hunger as well. Some of these people are hungry from the time they get up in the morning to the time they retire at night. It's almost as though they've passed the craving stage and have become gluttons. Others, such as binge eaters, may have no symptoms at all until their resistance is lowered due to stress. Then the cravings return, full force.

No one has yet defined why cravings are symptomatic of a fungus infection of the gastrointestinal tract. They could result from some effect on the central nervous system, or

DOES THIS CHAPTER RELATE TO *YOUR* CRAVINGS?

If your answer is yes, place a check by the item.

1. Have you ever taken birth control pills for more than one year? ( )
2. Have you ever taken antibiotics or cortisone for a long period (several months or more)? ( )
3. Do you crave sugar, chocolate, breads, and cheese or alcoholic beverages? ( )
4. Do you frequently have constipation or diarrhea or an upset stomach? ( )
5. Have you ever had frequent ear and throat infections? ( )
6. Have you ever suffered frequent bladder or vaginal *Monilia* infections? ( )
7. Have you been troubled by premenstrual tension or other menstrual problems? ( )
8. Have you experienced a loss of sexual desire? ( )
9. Do the fumes of chemicals such as gasoline, cleaning solutions, detergents, perfumes, after-shave lotions, etc., bother you? ( )
10. Do you frequently suffer from depression, poor memory, nervousness, fatigue, or poor concentration? ( )
11. Do you frequently get hives or rashes? ( )
12. Do you have a low pain threshold, evidenced by frequent headaches, or joint pains? ( )
13. During any pregnancies, were you sick often? ( )
14. Have you been told you have hypoglycemia, or do you suspect you have it? ( )

If you answered yes to seven or more questions, it's reasonable to suspect that you have candidiasis.

If you answered yes to ten or more questions, you should be checked by a doctor for the disease.

they might be a signal from the gastrointestinal tract. But there is no doubt that this condition simulates hunger. Any unusual, low-grade sensation in the gastrointestinal tract may be misinterpreted as hunger, causing one to eat more. Food will insure a short period of satisfaction, but as soon as the food moves down the gastrointestinal tract, the hunger returns.

Focal infections and cravings

Focal infection means that a particular location in our body is chronically infected. There may or may not be symptoms at the site of the infection, but there are often symptoms at various distant sites. Not much has been written about focal infections as a cause of symptomatic cravings.

Much of the material in medical literature 100 years ago dealt with the problems of focal infections and their ramifications. This idea is only now being rediscovered. Here's a quote from a book written by a doctor more than 50 years ago: "I have had several cases of blindness in one eye, in which the sight was completely restored by removing an offending area of focal infection."

If an infection starts in a mucous membrane such as those that line the respiratory tract, it may in some direct or indirect way lower the total resistance of the body. It may produce toxins that adversely affect our immune system, and allergic symptoms may even develop. When bacteria or fungi are infecting a membrane such as the mouth or nose, that inflamed membrane becomes more sensitive to allergens such as dust and pollen. This sensitivity further lowers the resistance of the body, and mineral imbalances occur. When there are relative mineral deficiencies, there will be changes in appetite. This progression of events creates a domino effect that eventually reaches the hunger centers. Although we don't know the exact chemical mechanisms that make this occur, we do know that for many patients, curing a focal infection has stopped the cravings.

The most common areas where focal infections reside are the mouth and gastrointestinal tract. It is not uncommon for a dentist to report that when a tooth is pulled, a patient reports a lessening of arthritis and other symptoms. The thought, of course, is that the infected tooth is creating a toxin that is affecting other organs of the body. Before the advent of antibiotics, the main cause of focal infections was bacteria. As antibiotics became more effective in destroying bacterial foci, one could reasonably conclude that this problem would be solved. It turns out, however, that when bacteria are destroyed, fungi grow, and so consequently you exchange one infection for another. As we will see later in this chapter, we now have an epidemic of focal yeast infections.

It's interesting that one of the major symptoms experienced in the gastrointestinal tract is hunger, and that the gastrointestinal tract can also be a primary area of infection. The stomach and intestines could be described as a culture tube thirty feet long. When cut and spread, its surface is about that of a tennis court. It's an enormous area loaded with media favorable to the rapid growth of immense colonies of germs. Since it is a sewer system of the body, a seething, fermentative process is continually going on. When this fermentation gets out of control, there is no doubt that it has the means of intoxicating the rest of the body. It would be very hard to deny what goes on in the digestive tract. Its sensations and health or the lack of health should have some effect on our eating habits.

The knowledge gap

There are many gaps in medical knowledge, and a certain amount is lost from generation to generation. New concepts force the retirement of old ones even though they may have been valid. In the interest of staying current, physicians have cast aside a number of valuable concepts.

Lost in the shuffle

For example, in the Inca civilization, rock cutting reached such an advanced level that there were techniques for slicing rock into precise cubes. Today, no one knows how the Incas practiced that craft. It was not done with chisels, for there are no chisel marks on the rocks. Possibly they had a method of melting the rock, perhaps with hot wires that were pulled through like a cheese cutter.

When the Spaniards came to South America and overpowered the Incas, there are no reports that the conquerors ever observed the rock cutting. This incredible feat, the slicing of rock to build temples, has been totally lost to our generation.

The same is true in medicine. When new treatments like antibiotics are discovered, old and effective treatments are downplayed to the new generations of doctors, and many good techniques are abandoned. In the 1800s, a focus of infection in an area such as the gastrointestinal tract was commonly found to cause symptoms at distant sites—in any organ of the body. With the advent of antibiotics, that concept was gradually cast aside. It is now being rediscovered by the allergists.

Gastrointestinal symptoms of candidiasis

Candida may invade the tissues of the gastrointestinal tract anywhere along the tract, from the mouth to the rectum. In the mouth, a coating of the tongue often appears and perhaps white spots on the gums or at the corners of the mouth. Candidiasis of the mouth is called thrush. Sometimes the only symptom is that the gums are sore, or they tingle, or the tongue has an unusual sensation. The symptoms are more obvious in children. In adults, they tend to be less distinct.

A little farther down in the esophagus, the symptoms may appear as frequent heartburn or a tendency to belch and regurgitate. If the stomach is affected, there may be indigestion or the feeling of a sour stomach. Very often the individual suffers from constipation, sometimes alternating with diarrhea, or there may be just diarrhea. If we develop gas, distension, or pains, we may suspect an ulcer.

In the lower abdomen there is often a cramping sensation combined with swelling or distension of the stomach after eating, as well as growling and gurgling sounds. Because of chronic constipation, hemorrhoids or itching may develop in the rectal area. Mucus or blood in the stool is rarely a problem.

Respiratory symptoms of candidiasis

A few of the more severely infected patients give off a foul odor or a peculiar smell because they breathe the yeast out into the air as they exhale. There may be swelling around the eyes as well as a swelling of the face.

A number of people eventually get symptoms similar to an allergy such as runny nose, sneezing, stuffiness, and post-nasal drip or a chronic cough. These symptoms may occur at different times of the day, very often early in the morning. Asthma also may occur. It's easy for *Candida* to get into the sinuses and produce chronic sinusitis. Changes in the mucous membrane, occurring as a result of the fungus, make it easy to develop bacterial or viral diseases. Very often, with just the slightest change in health, the person can experience a sore throat, an earache, pneumonia, or bronchitis. When antibiotics are prescribed to get rid of the bacteria, the fungus will be able to take advantage once again.

Symptoms of candidiasis on the skin

Because the hormonal system is disturbed, the skin may be drier than usual or even scaly, and skin diseases such as acne will flare up. There may be skin rashes, hives, eczema, chronic skin blemishes, and itching. Many candidiasis victims have an embarrassing problem with smelly feet and underarms. They may now notice for the first time some fungus growth on the skin or the nails.

Candidiasis and menstruation

Candidiasis frequently causes menstrual disturbances such as changes in flow and cycle. Cramping and premenstrual symptoms may also develop. It's not unusual for patients to experience a salty or metallic taste in their mouths and to smell unpleasant odors. Or there may be some loss of taste or smell. An occasional woman may notice that she feels lightheaded or dizzy before her period. Perhaps she suffers a mild hearing loss. Other patients complain of noises being too loud. Night blindness or other vision changes such as blurring also occur. One of the most common premenstrual problems is a feeling of clumsiness. It is possible that when one has these symptoms a severe *Candida* infection is present, causing the senses to miscalculate the distance or location of objects. The mechanism by which the infection causes these neurological problems is explained in Chapter 11 on premenstrual cravings.

There may or may not be a decreased interest in sex, and sometimes personality changes occur, resulting in bizarre emotions and depression. Sufferers can become irritable, nervous, excited, or anxious. There may be problems with concentration, memory, and with reasoning. And very often the person loses her normal self-confidence and develops a sense of helplessness.

These problems most often occur in women of childbearing age who have reported vaginal symptoms such as discharge. Vaginal itching can also occur, even without a discharge.

There may be some soreness around the vagina, accompanied by burning and itching. Scratching in response to the irritation may cause secondary bacterial infections to occur. Many women also suffer bladder problems, both frequency of and burning on urination. If the women are treated with antibiotics, the yeast infection is often encouraged. This is one reason why many women have bladder infections that never seem to disappear.

Weight gain due to water retention is also a common complaint. Many times, coincidentally, these so-called chronic bladder problems develop after pregnancy, at a time when the yeast tends to be in its fullest growth.

Musculoskeletal symptoms of candidiasis

When the musculoskeletal system is affected, there may be stiffness in the joints, a feeling of incipient arthritis. Sometimes the joints may actually become inflamed. These symptoms are especially acute before a rain or damp weather, when the mold spores are most prevalent.

Neurological symptoms and candidiasis

Even the brain is not exempt from yeast toxins. The toxins and byproducts of yeast are released into the bloodstream, then flow throughout the body, irritating the most sensitive organs in the individual.

Candidiasis can cause loss of memory and the ability to concentrate. The victim will frequently enter a room in the house, then forget why she went; she only knows she feels foggy and "spaced out." Changes in sleep pattern can occur, causing either insomnia or the need for excessive sleep.

When the body is saturated with toxins, the result can be a feeling of "not being right" and of just plain exhaustion. Other common symptoms include migraine, sinus or tension headaches, depression, anxiety, and uncontrollable crying.

Chemical allergies as a major symptom of candidiasis

Many physicians familiar with candidiasis believe that when full-blown, it greatly increases susceptibility to chemical allergens, both those ingested in foods and inhaled chemicals such as colognes, exhaust fumes, and hair spray. Cigarette smoke seems to particularly trouble these people. Even the smell of newspaper print can cause sensitive people to suffer personality changes or exhaustion, to the point of falling asleep while reading the paper. Hand contact with chemicals (detergents, chlorine, soaps) also causes reactions.

It's hard to know whether problems with the chemicals or foods are really allergies or simply intolerances, since the body loses much of its ability to resist and handle foreign substances when it is full of toxins.

Hypochondriac or not

Personality changes are a visible result of constant reactions to the environment. When we ask patients if they've ever been considered a hypochondriac, many say yes. Their problems can easily be mistaken if the doctor is not aware that a chemically allergic person is constantly having reactions beyond his control.

What triggers candidiasis?

Candida albicans infection, like all diseases, develops in response to a number of triggering events that act strongly to stimulate yeast growth. Refer to the questions in the box on page 104. Answering "yes" to selected questions may strongly suggest candidiasis. In general, circumstances that foster the disease are:

1. The constant or frequent abuse of chocolate, sugar, colas, breads, pastas (Mexican and Italian food), cheeses, wine, beer
2. A major trauma or stress including economic disturbances, a death, loss of job, health problems, and family breakups
3. Fatigue from overwork or overworry

If these problems occur simultaneously, they are likely to weaken our resistance. Our ability to ward off disease is a sign of good health. In a weakened condition, the body can be successfully attacked by bacteria and fungus.

Bacteria and yeast in the colon: The dynamic duo

Bacteria and fungi grow naturally in the colon. It's a symbiotic relationship. These organisms help us with our bodily processes, and we let them live peacefully. Since fungi and bacteria both need nourishment, they learn to share available food to coexist. If we ingest antibiotics to kill bacteria that have invaded, let's say, our ears, the antibiotics travel throughout all parts of our body. They can't discriminate between "good" and "bad" bacteria, so they destroy them all, including much-needed "friendly" bacteria. All food now goes to the fungi, who feast and grow. Wherever they are, they spread. Women who get throat infections and take antibiotics often note a subsequent vaginal *Monilia* infection, which then requires an antifungal agent to bring relief.

Where do the toxins form?

When the body tries to defend itself against yeast, our antibodies lock together with the yeast. This complex can then circulate in our blood and interfere with the activities of various enzymes and the metabolic processes of our hormonal and nervous systems.

It's of interest to note that each patient has different symptoms at different times, according to which combination of tissues is involved. The degree of irritation can also vary widely.

Stress as a trigger to candidiasis. The number one triggering agent is stress. Most people suffer stress sooner or later, and often the stress is severe. If the right circumstances occur together—for example, overeating of the wrong foods combined with illness or overwork—the fungus may begin to spread and cause symptoms.

Pregnancy, a normal event, can be potentially stressful, especially if other problems such as nutritional or hormonal imbalance are present at the same time. One symptom of such imbalance is that the patient does not feel ''well.'' Another symptom is gaining a lot of weight or accumulating excessive water in the tissues.

Cortisone as a trigger to candidiasis. In addition to antibiotics, another triggering agent is the overuse of cortisone. Adults with collagen diseases, bone and muscle diseases, and some metabolic diseases are sometimes given cortisone or other anti-inflammatory agents. If used for an extended period, this treatment can encourage fungus to grow.

The diet as a trigger to candidiasis. If the patient has a number of cravings, this may also indicate a yeast problem,

---

FOODS AND BEVERAGES THAT CONTAIN FUNGUS SPORES

Soy sauce	Mushrooms
Mayonnaise	Mushroom soup
Vinegar	Salad dressings
Beer and wine	Pickles
Whiskey	Baked goods
Gin	Olives
Most cheeses	Catsup
Malted products	Mince pie
Fruit juices—frozen, canned	Tomato sauce
Dried fruits	Milk fortified with vitamins

---

because that patient is probably consuming a great deal of sugar. Anyone who takes in large amounts of junk food is susceptible to the expansion of yeast colonies, especially during times of stress.

This brings to mind certain ethnic groups who frequently eat pasta or other starchy foods. Two good examples would be those of Italian and Hispanic origin. There have been no studies addressing this matter specifically, but my personal experience with Hispanic patients has shown them to have frequent and definite cravings for bread and cheese. In my estimation, most Hispanics are either allergic-addicted (see Chapter 6) or have candidiasis.

Refined sugars may cause symptoms in several ways:

1. They feed the yeast cells living in your digestive tract, causing them to multiply.
2. They upset the insulin/sugar balance in your blood, creating hypoglycemia, which puts a stress on the body and thus leads to easier development of disease.
3. The sugars in large amounts act like a drug, not a food, and upset the neurological system.
4. Sugars overutilize the nutritional supplies both through overusage and by altering the mineral ratios.

5. They may upset the acid-base balance which influences enzyme activity.
6. If you are allergic to them, the reaction puts stress on the body.

Overeating pasta, bread and cheese may not in itself cause mold growth (some say it does, others say it doesn't), but it can encourage it. Many pasta-related foods and junk foods contain sugar in amounts stimulatory to the yeasts.

Environmental mold as a triggering agent. Overexposure to mold can lead to an overpowering of the immune system. An overload can occur when we eat mold-yeast in our bread and cheeses and live in an environment where considerable mold is present.

Mold is everywhere, indoors and outdoors. It's primarily found in damp, dark places like basements and cellars, but it grows in other places too: in the dampness of a shady garden area, around our sinks and on the bathroom walls, in closets, under our rugs, and even in our pillows (if the pillow contains foam rubber). Everyone knows the reactions that airborne mold spores can have on the respiratory tract. We also know that allergists are forever trying to desensitize people against such molds.

Mold spores survive underground; when released, they float in the air like pollen. They grow outdoors on almost any decomposing matter such as leaves, rubber, wood, or paper, and they can also grow on normal vegetation.

A therapist may ask a patient to look for sources of mold around the home, such as damp basements, bathrooms, closets, drawers, hampers, mattresses, carpets, upholstered furniture, pillows, rags, sleeping bags, old magazines, books, newspapers, flowerpots, poorly ventilated kitchens, certain areas of the wallpaper, fruits and vegetables stored in basements, and shaded areas of the lawn and garden which tend to retain moisture.

Birth control pills as a triggering agent. The birth control pills contain synthetic progesterone. This hormone changes the vaginal lining in a way that makes it easier for yeasts to grow. When synthetic progesterone is given to a patient, not only can vaginitis occur, but yeasts may grow in the gastrointestinal tract as well.

It is common for women to report ill health after starting birth control pills, but when the pills are discontinued, the ill health often persists. It may have started a candidiasis problem that, once begun, continues to proliferate. For some reason, estrogen prescribed for women during menopause does not seem to encourage yeast growth.

How we test for candidiasis

The object of tests is to prove the presence of a particular microorganism—in this case, the fungus. There are three types of tests: cultures, antibody tests, and skin tests.

First, we take samples from an infected area and place them in a test tube or dish containing a culture medium. The object is to see whether the organism will then grow on this special medium; at that point we can identify it.

We may also check the blood for antibodies. The presence of antibodies reveals that our immune system has responded to an infection. It doesn't always tell whether the infection is past or present.

Third, we can do skin tests. Again, positive findings don't indicate the time frame of an infection unless a previous test was negative. Like many tests, skin tests are not completely accurate.

Another way of diagnosing a patient's problem is to do a therapeutic drug trial. We give the patient an antifungal medicine to kill the fungus. If improvement occurs, then we may have made the correct diagnosis. This particular diagnostic technique was used long before present laboratory tests were used. It has been useful to physicians for hundreds of years.

Candida albicans is an ornery devil, and it's difficult for any of these lab tests to be on target in their diagnosis. Because *Candida albicans* grows in everyone, antibodies against it also exist in all of us. Occasionally, a series of tests showing rising antibody levels are of help. Most doctors feel that a good history and a clinical trial, along with an elimination diet, are about the only accurate ways of determining whether this disease is present or not.

It's not "all in your head"

Many times patients will not even mention their symptoms to their family doctor because they assume the response will be negative. They know they are going to be told the same old cliché: "It's all in your head." Yet they know intuitively that their problem is real and become frustrated when trying to communicate. Often they prefer to conceal their symptoms, rather than to go through another barrage of "get hold of yourself" or that infuriating "knowing look."

Understandably, it's difficult to diagnose and treat a disease that seems to fluctuate over time and may vary from one organ to the next. For candidiasis is a disease with an array of seemingly unrelated symptoms, all of which constantly change according to the combination of organs involved. It's a diagnostician's nightmare, a never-ceasing challenge in the ongoing struggle against the wily "man-eating" plant.

If you think that the fungus among us is getting the best of you, don't despair. You'll find methods of treatment in the next chapter.

CHAPTER EIGHT

Treating Yeast-Related Cravings

Monilia is not in any way a part of the human body. It's a foreign substance, and the human body reacts to organisms that are unfamiliar. Many strange, minute life forms attack our bodies daily. We continually encounter fungi, viruses, and bacteria, so we would be constantly ill if we did not have a way of fending off these attackers.

THE IMMUNE SYSTEM: OUR FIRST LINE OF DEFENSE

Fortunately, we have a protective mechanism called the immune system. At the present time there is a great interest in that system, for we are learning more and more each year as a result of the research efforts in the field of cancer and AIDS.

First, some general facts about the immune system. We know, for example, that it has a number of things in common with the neurological and endocrine systems. All three work through the same enzymes and the same proteins, and the cells of these systems are actually quite similar. Things that affect the immune system often affect the endocrine, or hormone, system and the neurological system as well. We know that behavioral changes can affect the immune system and, conversely, that immune disregulation can affect behavior. I bring this to your attention because these close interrelationships are the cause of so many diverse and seemingly unrelated symptoms caused by candidiasis.

We know that social aberrations in our present society may be affecting our immune systems. We also know that these changes can ultimately affect the genetic pool, as more and more people with inferior immune systems populate society.

Immunity: The front lines

When a foreign substance attacks our body, our immune system responds by becoming stronger. Most of the time the immune system wins and we recover—but not always. Sometimes the attacker persists, and we reach a point of standoff.

The first defenders to appear when the body is invaded are the white blood cells, or leukocytes. These cells have various functions. Like scouts in a regular army, one group of these cells has the function of deciding whether the cell or material they come in contact with is normal or a foreign substance that has potential for causing harm. They then identify these cells so that other white blood cells (killer cells) can destroy them.

We also have suppressor cells. These suppressor cells regulate the killer cells so that they do not attack our own body by mistake. They are responsible for making sure that the killer cells can discriminate between foreign cells and our own. Certain diseases called autoimmune diseases occur when the suppressor cells do not function well and the killer cells turn and attack our own bodies. Some scientists suspect this process may also be one of the mechanisms of aging.

Toxins: Where do they come from?

Your vulnerability to disease depends upon the health of your immune system. Some white blood cells simply destroy invaders, but others produce antibodies that neutralize them. The neutralized invader becomes a toxin that the body has to get rid of; when there are a lot of these particles in our blood, we are said to be toxic. When waste products from germs accumulate at higher and higher levels, this rising load of toxins has a paralyzing effect on the white blood cells.

High toxin levels make a person feel ill, and various symptoms result. Treatment reduces these toxins to the lowest point possible in order to heal the person and to unlock the immune system and give it a chance to get back in control.

Toxins go for the weakest spot

If a person has a tendency toward psoriasis, for example, the toxins will irritate the skin's diseased cells and stir up symptoms. If the person has a weakness in the kidney area, kidney cells will be the first attacked by the toxins. If the patient has a problem related to obesity and hunger, the toxins may stir up excessive hunger and cravings.

The antigen connection

An antigen is defined as a substance that stimulates an immune response from the body. This stimulation causes the white blood cells to produce antibodies. The antibody, as you recall, is the material that neutralizes foreign substances. *Candida albicans* has many antigens—at least 79. Our immune system is responsible for taking care of them. Since there are so many antigens and they are different in each individual, it's difficult for the body to defend against all of them. Even worse, if there is some inherited inability to respond, the individual will succumb to the invasion.

Some people have all the luck

When a new flu virus appears, the population is not prepared for it. People do not have inborn genetic virus antibodies that can combat a new virus strain, and therefore they get influenza over and over again. In addition, we have even less ability to fight yeast infections than viruses. Those who are prone to repeated yeast invasions often have an inherited weakness. It's indicative of yeast's survivability that it has such a tenacious and voracious appetite for humans who have little resistance to it. Certain families in our society have incredibly poor resistance to fungus.

Individuals with chronic yeast infections apparently have an immunological unresponsiveness. Therefore the antigen is tolerated by the tissues and is not completely rejected by the body. Because it is not rejected, it grows steadily, and the toxins reach other areas of the body and affect any systems that are weak.

Stalemate

The very fact that someone does have a chronic yeast infection means that person's immune system is partially paralyzed. When the immune system starts to tolerate the presence of a foreign invader, then we have something known as a stalemate. In wartime, armies opposing each other reach a stalemate, and neither can make any progress. In the First World War, there was trench warfare, where neither army could claim victory. For years, the front lines stayed at an impasse. In more recent times, in both the Korean and the Vietnam wars, the front lines often did not change much for months or years at a time.

The stalemate phenomenon in our immune system can be demonstrated in other chronic infections and can also be produced experimentally in animals. It's been seen, for example, in leprosy and in certain stages of tuberculosis. We can reach a stalemate at many different stages of fungus infection. It can occur on the surface of our body when the mold first invades, or after molds have invaded our tissues to greater extent.

When these poisons first flood our bloodstream, we are able to resist them. But at some point it seems the load becomes too great and the body is less able to handle these toxins. It may be that our defense system is one of the first systems to be harmed by the toxins. When stalemate has been produced experimentally in animals, it often can be reversed quickly by treating the area where the infection started. This quickly decreases the waste products and stops the toxins from paralyzing the animal's defense systems.

A good example of this phenomenon occurs in the monilial vaginal infections commonly seen in women. Often, early episodes of acute vaginitis clear up without treatment or with minor medication. With age, however, there seem to be more recurrences of these infections, and sometimes the condition becomes chronic. As time passes, the women become more or less immune to drugs, and they eventually just reconcile themselves to living with the condition.

The benefits of treatment

Probably one of the most beneficial results of this treatment is to restore normal hormone function. Abnormalities of menstrual bleeding and severe premenstrual changes, as well as the woman's mental state, tend to improve. Often sex drive increases, and the skin exhibits a finer smoothness because the hormones are now better able to affect the skin positively. Acne may clear up, skin lesions improve, headaches may decrease, bladder problems become less common, and there's an increase in energy and vitality.

The mental state of the individual may improve remarkably, with improvement in memory and concentration as uncontrollable emotions, moodiness, and reaction to food allergies tend to diminish. *One of the first and most important symptoms to vanish is hunger and cravings*. It's a sure and important sign of progress.

HOW TO FIGHT BACK

By now you understand a great deal about the problem of gastrointestinal yeast infections, and you're probably wondering what can be done about it.

How yeasts are treated

If you have these cravings as a result of *Candida albicans* you will never really stop craving until you have been properly treated. The following suggestions are useful, but they don't take the place of a medical treatment program.

Finding out more

First, learn more about the problem. Here are two books that are a must:

The Yeast Connection
Wm. G. Crook, M.D.
Professional Books
P.O. Box 3494
Jackson, TN 38301

The Missing Diagnosis
Dr. Oren Truss
P.O. Box 26508
Birmingham, AL 35226

You can probably purchase Dr. Crook's book at local bookstores. You will have to contact Dr. Truss's office to order his book. I would urge you to do that if you suspect a serious problem as a result of candidiasis.

Change your diet

Why do we use diet to treat candidiasis? Why not just medicine? We use diets in candidiasis for the same reasons that diets are used in diabetes, hypoglycemia, hypertension, gout, and many other diseases. Certain foods can aggravate certain diseases. You certainly would not expect an individual who is allergic to milk to continue drinking it while you are attempting to build up that person's resistance. It would be a lot smarter to wait until the body is prepared to tolerate milk before resuming consumption.

Certain foods encourage yeast growth. By depriving the yeast of nutrients, one can slow down and inhibit its growth. Medicine can then do its job more effectively.

Diet is not the *treatment* for candidiasis. Do not think that simply because your symptoms improve, you have cured the disease. The fungus will survive and lie dormant and will continue to create toxic products, but on a slower scale. Diets prevent further growth—but they do not destroy the fungus. Conversely, if you do not improve with the diet, that doesn't mean that you do not have the disease. It simply may be that passive methods are not effective enough to solve the problem. Yeasts don't do as well with diets high in fat and protein; rather, they thrive on carbohydrates. Stopping the intake of sweets and starches prevents their further growth.

Do you get gas?

Patients with *Candida* often notice an increase in stomach gas or bloating after eating foods that contain mold. This includes breads, pastries, mushrooms (which are a fungus), aged cheeses, and alcohol (especially beer and wine). If you are taking yeast tablets, stop them at once, and avoid all fermented liquids, such as vinegar.

The importance of the diet

Mold will attack anything that was originally alive. Small amounts are found on almost all foods that have been left out for even a short time. There is no diet that is entirely mold free, but reducing the amount of the mold in food restricts *Monilia* growth.

A diet is more important at the beginning of treatment than later, and many of these items can be reinstated in your diet after treatment is completed. Don't feel deprived; think of yourself as merely postponing the enjoyment of these good things until they are no longer a problem to your body. If your cravings are not overly severe, it's possible that the treatment might be effective within only a few weeks. If the problem is more complex, it will take longer.

Occasional departures from the diet aggravate some patients' cravings. In others, it doesn't seem to make much difference, so long as the deviation from the diet is not too frequent. It is the continuous intake of large amounts of offending foods that causes problems.

The diet can help in many ways

The diet helps in other ways, for many patients are allergic to corn, wheat, and other grains, especially malt. So the diet is beneficial to those who are food allergic-addicted.

Some patients who have mild to moderate hypoglycemia will also benefit from the diet. For hypoglycemics, the diet stops the overstimulation of the pancreas by carbohydrates. This can decrease weight, decrease hunger, and decrease cravings. We can't eliminate yeast-containing foods entirely, but we can consume them in the lowest possible amounts, long enough for our immune system to recover.

Patients with special problems

Patients who are chemically sensitive may find it much harder to alter their diet. Unfortunately, many of these people are intolerant of proteins. Since we are eliminating most of the foods they can tolerate, we must compensate. Sometimes these patients are better able to tolerate carbohydrates than protein. If so, we recommend complex starches (not sugars) until they improve. These variations are the reason why full treatment, if needed, should be monitored by a physician who is knowledgeable in this field.

Children should be taken off cow's milk and given goat's milk, and the rest of their diet adjusted accordingly. And remember, many vitamins and minerals contain yeast, so it is important to work with your physician and educate yourself in all these areas.

Diet for severe cravers

The first rule is to avoid all *simple* sugars such as:

table sugar	sucrose	glycogen	galactose
corn sugar	glucose	lactose	beet sugar
fructose	maltose	mannitol	date sugar

These are found in cakes, pies, donuts, candy, rolls, and cereals. Any sugar under any name, including "natural" sugars, must also be avoided:

honey	dried fruits
maple sugar	candied fruits
molasses	

Fast foods often contain added sugar, as do many if not most "innocent" prepackaged items such as soups, chicken slices, and so-called diet dinners. Read the labels.

What about fruit?

In general it's best to eat very little fresh fruit—none for the first 60 to 90 days. After that, stay mostly with apples, melons, and grapefruit. Fruits are pure sugar, and even though they contain good fiber along with vitamins and minerals, they do contribute to yeast growth.

The second group of foods that encourage yeast are milk products, because the lactose in milk becomes sugar in the body:

whole milk	buttermilk
low-fat milk	sour cream
ice cream	yogurt

Cheeses are a problem because they are derived from milk and they also contain yeast. So eliminate:

swiss cheese	roquefort and other moldy
cottage cheese	cheeses
processed cheese food	cheese snacks
	macaroni and cheese

A third group of problem foods contains yeast and items that encourage yeast growth:

mustard	monosodium	boxed foods	sprouts
pickles	glutamate	containing	baker's yeast
soy sauce	(MSG)	yeast	mayonnaise
vinegar	sauerkraut	nuts that	salad dress-
enriched	mushrooms	seem	ing
foods	canned foods	to have a	smoked
peanuts and	containing	film of	meats
peanut but-	yeast	mold	brewer's
ter		horseradish	yeast
pistachios		mincemeat	
catsup			

The fourth group consists of liquids that stimulate yeast or decrease yeast resistance:

wine	gin	whiskey	instant coffee
rum	liqueurs	all regular	and tea
vodka	cider	coffee and	beer
herb teas	diet colas	tea	fruit juices
malted drinks	brandy		(all of them)

With a list like this, it might seem as though there is nothing left to eat, but read on:

Proteins You Can Have

beef	rabbit	lamb	most fish
pork	duck	quail	all shellfish
chicken	cornish hen	veal	eggs
turkey	tuna	game birds	

Beverages You Can Have

vegetable juices
bottled water

Bakery Products You Can Have

Cereals, grains, and bread that are without sugar or honey and are not made with yeast—that means checking labels carefully.

Vegetables You Can Have

Vegetables, including whole grains, are generally yeast free, but avoid corn and popcorn if you crave sugar because they encourage sugar cravings.

Diet for the less severe cravers

Avoid all sugar and sweets
Avoid cheese and yeast-baked bread
Avoid vinegar and mushrooms
Avoid caffeine-containing drinks: coffee, tea, some colas
Avoid alcohol, wine, and beer

Use the supplements recommended in this book to stay on the diet. After 10 to 20 weeks you can carefully test the waters to see if you can tolerate some of the foods you originally eliminated from your diet.

Second thoughts

Some doctors do not agree that diet plays a role in recovery from infection. I personally believe the three most important items to eliminate, if possible, are (1) sugar and all sugar-containing products, (2) all caffeine-containing products, and (3) alcohol of any type. Not forever, of course, but be very careful for at least two weeks. Then, if you break the rules, you will probably be able to tell if it made a difference by the symptoms you develop. You'll then know why the diet plays such an important role in candidiasis treatment.

Vitamin supplements

You may wish to use my technique. If so, use a yeast-free, sugar-free multivitamin and mineral once a day and 50 mg

B_6 three times daily. You can usually get these at health food stores.

For cravings, you can use 7½ grain alfalfa tablets—four each time the cravings start or at least four times daily. You may want to use niacinamide in 50 mg tablets to support the alfalfa. Be sure you review the material in Chapter 4. Use 2000 to 4000 mg vitamin C in the powdered form every two hours till the cravings stop. A combination of vitamin C and the Chapter 4 minerals will give total relief in almost all cases, but be aware that you must work out your own frequency schedule.

Some patients have reported to me that their cravings stopped after using caprylic acid. Take two to four 100 mg tablets every three hours until the cravings stop, then decrease the dosage to two tablets three times a day. Caprylic acid is often combined with other nutrients to make it more effective. Some health food stores carry the product but many don't. Allergy Research Group (P.O. Box 489, San Leandro, CA 94577, [415] 639-4572) sells a product called Caprylate Plus that I have found very effective.

The essential fatty acids mentioned in Chapter 3 are the last and most important nutritional ingredient. Your body needs gamma-linolenic acid to normalize many of the enzyme systems in the body. It will help correct the dry skin problem that many patients with *Candida* report.

If your balance of nutrients is poor, you are walking a tightrope, and a good breeze could blow you over. It's not the wind's fault; you're just perched too precariously for your own good. In a sense you're out on a limb because of your lack of good nutrition. Your chemical imbalance plus your genetic makeup has made you weak in some area.

How is your digestion?

Next we have to be sure you're digesting and assimilating your nutrients properly. Many doctors do tests for stomach acid and digestive enzymes. The inability to digest foods properly could be evidenced by frequent gas after meals, especially several hours later. To eliminate the gas, obtain tablets of bile salts and pancreatic enzymes from your local drugstore. Take two to four when you have gas to help you digest both your food and your vitamins.

If you are allergic to some foods on the diet but your allergy is relatively mild, then the food to which you are allergic-addicted may be taken in small amounts after three months of treatment. They also may be taken in larger amounts if you are using a rotational diet (see box). It is important not to overuse foods, because if they're used too often, your allergies start to redevelop.

Each doctor has a personal technique for reintroducing food to a patient. Most will attempt to get the patient back on as normal a diet as possible, to avoid malnutrition. We are able to tolerate a severely restricted diet for only a limited length of time.

BASIC RULES FOR A ROTATIONAL DIET

You can avoid overexposure and consequent development of food allergies by rotating the foods you eat. Allergists recommend this system for both prevention and treatment. Here are some basic rules.

1. Do not eat any food more than once every four days, even if you do not react to it.

2. Foods within the same family are likely to cause similar reactions. Check any food you react to against the food family list in this book. If your reaction is strong, do not use more than one food from that family every four days. You can ignore this rule if you are only mildly allergic to a food.

3. If you react to many different foods, keep your meals simple, with only one to three foods or food families.

4. Moderate servings are better than large servings for people who are strongly reactive.

5. Totally avoid any food you react to strongly for at least twelve weeks; then use it no more than twice a week.

Clean up your environment

The next problem is dealing with your environment. There are many molds found outside the body that have an ability to enhance *Monilia* infection. Any local area where there might be a large colony of mold spores will stimulate yeast growth within us. Mold grows well, for example, in basements, in older homes where water has been allowed to accumulate, in dry rot under rugs, in damp areas, in homes built near areas where the water drainage is poor, and in homes in highly humid areas.

In a few rare cases it might even be necessary for a person to move to a new residence. This may sound radical, but keep in mind that over the years, doctors have often advised allergic people to change climates.

It's important to keep your feet dry and to change your socks often if they get wet from exercise. Any area of the body where fungus can easily grow presents a problem. Especially vulnerable are housewives and bartenders, whose hands are always in water. Fungus growth on the body's surface prevents the internal treatment from working, so athlete's foot or other skin infections must be treated locally as well.

Drugs can aggravate the problem

If used at all during the treatment, antibiotics should be kept to a minimum. If they are necessary, especially in the case of children, one should combine them with drugs to prevent yeast growth. They can, in most cases, be safely taken together. It is important not to use antibiotics for minor problems such as acne. Discontinue antibiotics as soon as they are no longer needed, but *check with your physician first*, for stopping too soon can be dangerous.

Yeast growth often occurs in women who have chronic bladder problems. If you are getting antibiotics from another physician during the time of this treatment, it is important to inform the physician treating you for candidiasis that you are taking them. The same goes for all medications you are taking.

The next problem is birth control pills. Some women say they can't live with them and can't live without them. An alternative system of birth control must be worked out, if at all possible, during the treatment phase. Over a third of the women using these pills develop or intensify vaginal yeast infections. It is most likely that the yeast in the bowel is also encouraged to thrive.

Women who are pregnant should watch for signs of yeast infections, too. Anti-*Candida* medications may be used during pregnancy, since the medication does not actually enter the blood or affect the fetus.

Candida can be sexually transmitted, and sexually active women will undoubtedly have a yeast infection at some point. Precautions should be taken to avoid this along with other sexually transmitted diseases. Even kissing can lead to transmission of *Monilia*, especially tongue kissing, so keep that in mind when you're under the mistletoe.

Cortisone is used by physicians fairly often for allergy and skin diseases. However, many people try to avoid this drug because of its bad reputation. It is an excellent medicine, but not for patients with yeast problems, because it suppresses the immune system and allows yeast to grow rampantly. This decision should not be made by the patient; it's really up to the physician to weigh the pros and cons. If you are given cortisone by another doctor while you are in a treatment program, you should immediately inform the doctor who is treating you for candidiasis.

If a person must take cortisone for any reason, it would be good to complement it with an antifungal agent, especially if the patient is aware of fungus on any parts of the body.

There are other types of drugs, too, that encourage candidiasis. For example, immunosuppressants used before and after organ transplants and in the treatment of cancer and leukemia patients are especially troublesome. Unfortunately, such drugs are usually given to people who already are in a weakened state.

Physicians may add thyroid drugs or hormones to the *Candida* program if they feel the patient will benefit, but progesterone should be used guardedly. It has recently been used with some success prior to menstruation for treatment of PMS (premenstrual syndrome), but women should be aware that it can aggravate a *Candida* problem.

Using Nystatin to treat candidiasis

The drug Nystatin is sometimes used as a treatment for *Candida* infections. A word of caution. Although a family physician certainly can prescribe this drug, it is unlikely that a general practitioner will have had enough experience to use the drug properly. If it's not prescribed by an experienced practitioner, the treatment with Nystatin is likely to fail, not because the drug isn't effective, but because it requires adjustments in each individual, and not all doctors have that expertise. Some of the reasons for this are:

1. The entire gastrointestinal tract must be coated from the mouth to the rectum. This must be done several times each day.
2. The amount of medicine given to each patient varies according to the doctor's evaluation.
3. Clinically sensitive patients often overreact to the drug, causing an intensification of their symptoms. An improper dose in a chemically sensitive patient could provoke a crisis.
4. A few patients are not able to tolerate this drug at all, and substitute treatments must be used.

Another problem is getting the dosage adjusted for maximum effectiveness. Only a physician experienced with this drug knows how to deal with each change in the symptoms. He or she may want to increase or decrease the dosage. In some cases, the dosage may need to be extraordinarily high, and family physicians may be unaware of the safety factors involved. A general practitioner might not understand that the patient is being underdosed and that that is the reason why there has been no response to treatment. The doctor may mistakenly feel the treatment itself is ineffective and will prematurely abandon it.

Another problem for an inexperienced physician occurs when the patient becomes refractive to the treatment. The physician must have some idea of when to discontinue treatment and what to do if there's no response. It's not so much the differences between diseases but rather the variations in people that the physician must be concerned about. Some people react adversely to Nystatin tablets, and often the tablet coating is the cause of the problem.

The way in which Nystatin is administered is also important in the treatment. Sometimes it's taken orally, sometimes through the nose, sometimes in pill form, sometimes as a powder. These approaches may be different in different patients for various reasons. The physician should also be aware that there are other drugs that may support this drug and may be needed during the treatment. Certain food supplements also affect the results of the drug.

As emphasized, the actual treatment for candidiasis should be supervised by a physician who is knowledgeable and experienced in this disease and its treatment. It should not be undertaken by the patient alone and should probably not be administered by a physician who is unaware of the full range of the treatment program. Any interested physician may contact Dr. Oren Truss in Birmingham, Alabama.

Nystatin is safer than most of the other antifungal drugs, and other medication can be used intermittently with it. The drug can be valuable as a diagnostic tool as well as for therapy. It is not absorbed from the gastrointestinal tract and has no uses other than for yeast infections. It may also be applied on the skin or in the vagina.

Electron microscope studies have indicated that the yeasts get into the surface cells of the mucous membranes and remain inside. It is not as easy for drugs to attack the yeast cells when they're hidden inside body cells. The whole mechanism is not clearly understood, but the clinical results are important.

The object is to reduce the toxins released by yeast cells so the body's resistance system can recover its strength. We must bring this drug into contact with the greatest possible number of yeast cells, for when the encounter occurs it explodes them. How this is accomplished varies from person to person. Sometimes the drug has to be used in several forms simultaneously for maximum effectiveness. No food should be eaten for at least two hours after the drug is taken. All areas where the yeast is known to exist on the body should be treated simultaneously.

The drug itself produces almost no toxic reaction. Some supposed cases of drug reaction are actually caused by substances added in the manufacturing. Basically, the drug itself is extremely safe. It has been given in enormous doses to leukemia patients to control the spread of yeast. Usually it is possible to kill at least 80 percent of the yeast cells fairly rapidly, but the remaining 20 percent are extremely difficult to eradicate in all patients. Under the right circumstances, the yeast cells can multiply within hours or days to an almost uncontrollable number. However, if 80 percent of the yeast cells are killed in those initial few days and weeks, the toxins present are greatly reduced.

How many people can be helped by this therapy? Experienced therapists say 50 percent can be cured, 25 percent greatly improved, and the rest undecided. Nystatin only kills yeast, it does not aid the immune system.

Some cases have been cured within as little as six weeks, while others have taken as long as three years. This type of chronic infection can set people back years. Those taking this treatment should understand that their condition did not occur overnight, so they cannot expect to recover immediately. Some people improve rapidly in terms of symptoms, but their infection still exists for long periods.

How long should the person continue the treatment if there are no results? That, again, is up to the physician. Some patients will not recover on this program, but fortunately, a fairly large number with serious cases do get better. *Fortunately, also, at least 80 to 90 percent of those with cravings will have craving relief with this treatment, and in some cases, total cure.*

If patients taking Nystatin have relapses when it is discontinued, then they must be kept on it indefinitely. In certain cases, dosage might be increased, during times of stress. If the drug fails to work, then the doctor may have to use another drug.

Vaccines

Another treatment that seems to be effective in this disease is vaccine therapy. It is the same method used by allergists to treat pollen allergies.

Outstanding and often dramatic improvement can occur within a short time at the beginning of treatment, but vaccine therapy itself has some side reactions.

Getting better

Relief of symptoms usually occurs in this order: *The craving disappears first*; headaches, if they have been a symptom, are second to stop. The next common ailment that seems to be relieved is problems with the gastrointestinal tract, constipation or diarrhea. Fourth, the vaginitis disappears. Next, the nervous system stabilizes, and emotions are more in control. The next improvement is seen in behavior patterns; rebelliousness disappears, along with certain sadistic behavior. Finally, skin rashes begin to clear up.

Summing it up

Candida albicans is a fungus that can invade any mucous membrane in our body. It lives quietly in our bowels but tends to spread under certain circumstances.

Whatever the reason for growth, it can produce toxins which circulate through our body and cause serious disturbances. Many patients who have hidden *Candida* infections will manifest unexplained, difficult-to-diagnose symptoms.

One of the most prominent symptoms caused by the *Candida* infection is intense cravings for sweets, breads, and cheeses. This particular symptom is such a good marker for the disease that doctors use it to determine improvement—or lack of improvement—while their patients are in therapy. If the treatment is working, the cravings disappear. If the therapy isn't effective, the cravings come back. We have, therefore, a reliable way to deal with cravings. Relief has been reported by thousands of patients across the country. It works most of the time. It is believed this craving relief may be permanent, or at least effective for a long period.

The therapy that leads to this long-term improvement consists of a diet, avoidance of certain drugs, avoidance of some environments, good nutrition, and the antifungicide, Nystatin.

One other important point during the early treatment stages: In the time period before Nystatin or vaccines suppress cravings, one might try the supplements mentioned in Chapters 3 and 4. These vitamin-mineral supplements will have no effect on the treatment of candidiasis, but they will assist the patient in complying with the diet. They can thereafter be used to keep the patient from straying too far from the "straight and narrow."

If there is one word of advice that might be given to patients who believe they have this problem and are contemplating treatment, it would be this: *patience*. And the second most important thing is to give *full cooperation* to your physician, for an effective partnership is necessary to achieve optimum results.

PART FOUR

Special Craving Problems

CHAPTER NINE

Craving by the Clock

The theory that people eat to calm themselves has been a well-accepted psychological concept for many years. Common sense and personal experience seem to verify it. The original belief was that during times of stress, food would symbolically provide enough comfort to soothe and reassure the distressed individual.

However, as the biochemistry of the brain was studied further, it became apparent that there are physical reasons for food cravings. These changed beliefs involve the emerging science of *neurotransmitters*: chemicals involved in transmitting nerve impulses to and from the brain and throughout the body.

DEPRESSION, NEUROTRANSMITTERS, AND HORMONES
The new concept of biochemical cycles

Researchers Judith Wurtman, Ph.D., and Richard Wurtman, M.D., have studied individuals who crave on a 24-hour schedule. These cravers don't recognize the pattern because they may be nibbling at other times as well. But regardless

153

of other food intake, they always crave carbohydrates, usually some form of sugar, at the same time each day. The time of the day they experience cravings varies, because not all of them desire something sweet at, say, 8 P.M. every night. The pattern seems to be tied to the individual's circadian rhythm, an internal time clock. When the internal alarm goes off, it's time for sweets.

There's an old joke: What does a 500-pound parrot say? Answer: "Polly wants a cracker—NOW!" When a food alarm goes off, then "Polly wants a sweet—NOW." There's no sense of satisfaction until that urge is satisfied. If the need goes unfulfilled, irritability develops, followed by depression and moodiness.

Depression is indeed the major factor. Victims of cravings become moody and depressed if they don't have sugar. The depression is caused by a deficiency of a neurotransmitter called *serotonin*. For some unknown reason, levels of serotonin become low one or more times a day, always at precisely the same hour.

I'd like to clarify a point: Not everyone who likes to snack or nosh is a true craver. Actually, we have no idea just how many people crave carbohydrates on a cyclic basis. Even when people who crave rhythmically are identified, this group needs to be distinguished from those whose hunger is triggered by other mechanisms.

Our adrenal glands also turn off by the clock

Cortisone, a hormone produced by our adrenal glands, is possibly another cause of craving by the clock. It is well known that the production of cortisone by our adrenal glands waxes and wanes during a 24-hour period. In many people it becomes extremely low around 3 A.M. and 3 P.M., since the adrenal hormones that moderate blood sugar allow it to fall at these times. The fall in blood sugar leads to lack of energy, lack of concentration, irritability, and other symptoms. A snack containing sugar can quickly relieve these sensations. Remember the old Dr. Pepper commercials? "Dr. Pepper peps you up and gives you a lift at ten, two, and four"—common times of energy fadeout.

There is one big difference between cravings caused by cortisone deficiency and those that result from a lack of serotonin. The former causes cravings at *about* the same time each day, but a serotonin deficiency will ring the hunger bell at *exactly* the same time daily.

The food that relieves both depression and cravings

Those who crave carbohydrates at exactly the same time each day can't get relief from protein—only sugar will satisfy them. It seems their cravings are tied more to mood than to low energy. Since they suffer from depression, what they seek is mood elevation, and sweets seem to be the key. If any other type of food is taken along with the sweets, it spoils the sense of satisfaction and relief. There are reasons why this group of cravers needs just the right food.

How does a sugar fix block depression and cravings?

The events go in this order:

1. Serotonin is the brain chemical, or neurotransmitter, which when deficient often causes feelings of depression.
2. The body manufactures serotonin from a tiny protein particle, an amino acid called tryptophan.
3. Tryptophan comes from foods that contain protein, such as meat. After being digested and absorbed, it attaches itself to a blood protein called albumin and continues to circulate in the blood.
4. When sugar is eaten, it helps tryptophan get into the brain, where it is transformed into serotonin.
5. There, the serotonin relieves the depression.

Why you can't just eat protein and get the tryptophan you need

When foods containing protein are eaten, the food is broken down by the body. The protein is broken into smaller and smaller particles until it is reduced to amino acids. There are large amino acids as well as small ones. The brain needs amino acids for a variety of purposes. To reach their destination, they must compete for transport through a cellular membrane called the blood/brain barrier. If there aren't enough spaces on the transport system they can't all get through. Many of these large amino acids are more aggressive than tryptophan, so it often gets left behind. At that point, there's a reduction in serotonin, so the desired mood elevation is not forthcoming. One reason that tryptophan gets sidetracked is that it's usually not as plentiful in foods as other amino acids. The other large amino acids are present in such great numbers that tryptophan is overwhelmed. Mood change will not occur until a carbohydrate in concentrated form is absorbed.

Why? Because carbohydrates (sugar) help tryptophan get through the blood/brain barrier.

How does sugar make tryptophan relieve cravings?

Sugar helps tryptophan enter the brain by getting rid of the other amino acids. Concentrated sugar in the form of sweets stimulates the production and release of insulin from the pancreas. Insulin then forces the other amino acids out of the blood into cells. Tryptophan does not leave the blood with the others because it is attached to another blood amino acid—albumin.

Studies on the brains of rats show that after a high-protein meal, very little tryptophan gets into the brain, but after a carbohydrate meal, there is a definite rise in the brain's tryptophan level.

Special problems of the diabetic

One of the problems for individuals with the adult-onset type of diabetes is that the insulin needed to get the tryptophan into the blood works ineffectively. These patients are said to be insulin resistant. Because the insulin in their bodies can't get the job done, diabetics are forced to use larger amounts of sugar to gain the relief they seek. This inability to get enough relief from carbohydrates can lead to binge eating.

The effect on bulimics

Bulimics are people who alternately binge on large quantities of food and purge themselves by vomiting. They are affected by the same intense hunger as diabetics, and they may also have a need for immediate relief of depression. This can result in panic eating. After the attack, they fear the consequences of having devoured so much food, so they forcefully regurgitate in guilt, fear, and disgust. This overreaction disturbs both the person's psychology and physiology and begins a destructive cycle known as the binge/purge syndrome.

Diabetics who crave sugar do not get enough tryptophan into the brain to feel carbohydrate-full. Their need is like slow starvation. Bulimics, on the other hand, have a more intense need for immediate relief. Although some sufferers have disturbed or even psychotic personalities, the majority do not, and this leads us to believe that the attacks could be related to temporarily disturbed brain chemistry. Precisely what triggers these attacks has not been clearly defined.

Obesity

It's well known to professionals who treat overweight individuals that those who complete their weight loss often have rebound hunger. It's not uncommon for them to binge and have an immediate ten-pound gain. The reason for this is that after carbohydrate deprivation, it takes three times as much sugar to get tryptophan into the brain. Only then is serotonin made and satisfaction obtained.

There is another interesting relationship, as well. It's documented that amphetamines (appetite suppressants) will stop general hunger, but not cravings. There is one appetite suppressor, however, that is effective: Fenfluramine. This compound is known to increase serotonin levels.

What about the thin person?

A doctor in South Africa devised a method using rebound hunger to put weight on thin individuals who couldn't gain otherwise. He had them fast or diet until they lost five or ten pounds, then overeat until their weight was increased to five pounds beyond the starting point. He then had them fast or diet off those gained pounds, plus a little more. This increased their appetite to the point where they would overeat again until they were ten or more pounds over their original weight. Although the process was time-consuming, this take-off/put-on cycle was repeated until the subjects had successfully gained the desired weight. It should be noted that it's difficult to put weight on thin individuals with standard therapies.

Possible answers to some unanswered questions

1. *Why is it so hard to stay on a diet?* The reason could be due to a need for serotonin to elevate mood. Being deprived of carbohydrates while dieting leads to chronically low serotonin levels. This makes it easy to feel "down" while reducing, and the natural remedy is to eat.

2. *Why do people eat more when they get upset?* This reaction could be related to an immediate need for serotonin and mood elevation, especially for the overeater who prefers carbohydrates. It may be of interest to note that tryptophan has long been used as an antidepressant by some psychiatrists. There is another side to this, however; certain people lose their appetite when distressed. They are repelled by food. If they are forced to eat, their depression is not relieved. The person who doesn't want to eat during upsets apparently has

a different set of chemical mechanisms. Older textbooks on psychiatry often list loss of appetite as a sign of depression, apparently not recognizing that overeating during depression is just as common. Newer textbooks now list *change* in appetite as one sign of depression.

3. Doctors who treat overweight individuals often hear the question: *Why is it that after supper I never feel satisfied until I eat something sweet?* The answer is that it takes concentrated sugar in the form of a dessert to push tryptophan into the brain where it becomes serotonin. Serotonin then gives us the peaceful, quieted, relaxed feeling we seek.

4. It's known that weather affects eating patterns, and often more food is eaten in winter months than in summer. It used to be thought that the colder months increased caloric need and hence caused greater food intake. But it's now been discovered that there may be individuals who get more depressed during winter months. Dr. Rosenthal of the National Institute of Mental Health has called this condition *Seasonal Affective Disorder* (SAD). This type of depression seems to abate during the spring and summer and is more common in northern areas, where there is less sunlight. It should also be noted that the amount of light available is directly tied to the female menstrual cycle. This hormone cycle can be altered by changing the brightness or dimness of the environment.

Individuals with cyclic cravings often eat more during winter months. This may relate to a greater moodiness experienced at that time of the year. To keep things in perspective, in our chapter on yeast, we mention environmental mold count as being related to cravings. Damp weather increases mold count. In susceptible individuals, cravings increase. So you can see, there is a complexity of reasons why the craving phenomenon occurs.

TREATING CRAVINGS DUE TO LOW SEROTONIN

As we have said before, an ounce or two of sugar along with tryptophan will block this kind of clock cravings. So what kinds of carbohydrates (sugars) are best to use?

An ounce of sugar

Judith Wurtman, Ph.D., has written a book called *The Carbohydrate Craver's Diet* reporting research by her and her husband into cyclic cravings. In her book, she lists dozens of snacks containing small amounts of sugar that could be used to block carbohydrate cravings. It seems strange to prescribe sugar to relieve sugar cravings, but the concept is validated by the theory that using smaller, less problematic amounts will ensure control.

Dr. Wurtman's list of snacks includes three cups of popcorn, three ounces of jelly beans (shades of President Reagan), or several fig bars. To these snacks, tryptophan can be added in tablet form. Most health food stores or drugstores have 500 mg tryptophan tablets. The combination of a 100- to 200-calorie pure carbohydrate snack and tryptophan can relieve the cyclic craver's moodiness and depression quite effectively.

Keep in mind that the combination must be individually adjusted. I use different amounts of tryptophan with the snack. First I try a 500 mg tablet. Next I try one-and-a-half tablets, then two tablets, and soon up to three or four. Some psychiatrists have used doses as high as 1500 mg for treatment of depression. I'm cautious, though, about advising more than four tablets (2000 mg) because of possible side effects.

I've had patients complain of too much drowsiness, and others in whom increased serotonin led to headaches and irritability rather than relaxation. The common misconception that more is better should be avoided. I seek a balance, with the absolute lowest amount of substance that works. Everything that goes into the body has its effect. When chemical changes are intentionally created, they should be kept to a minimum.

Instead of snacks, I prefer to use a combination of tryptophan with vitamin B_6. This combination is useful for two reasons: First, it doesn't contain any calories, and second, it's more portable. You could try both approaches if you wish to see what works best. I use the tryptophan in different amounts, as previously mentioned, and to that I add various amounts of vitamin B_6. I prescribe a 50 mg B_6 tablet and then experiment with a quarter, a half, or a whole tablet. If that doesn't work, one can use one-and-one-half or two tablets with the tryptophan. That way we can cover everything from 12 mg to 100 mg to see what's most effective. I don't exceed 100 mg of B_6 at any one time, again because of the potential side effects. Too much B_6 can cause irritability, and when it has been used over a long period, neurological changes have been reported.

Another useful combination is tryptophan in the amounts mentioned, and niacinamide, 50 to 500 mg. Niacinamide is another factor that forces tryptophan into the brain. I've effectively used these items together when patients report cravings.

AFTER-DINNER SNACKING

Evening snacking

Wanting to eat something several hours after dinner seems to be extremely common. In my clinic more than 80 percent of those with weight problems report evening snacking. Most of them wish they could stop. Everyone recognizes that calories at bedtime can easily show up on one's stomach or hips.

Why do we eat in the evening? It's not hard to understand. An abundance of TV commercials stimulate the sensory organs. They don't call it prime time for nothing. Priming your pump for food is what's happening. Snacking in the evening is also a social nicety, a required amenity when one entertains; these nighttime nibbles provide an energy lift as well as enhancing camaraderie. It is also likely that some of those who have serotonin deficiencies develop them in the late evening.

It's not easy to stop

Some of the methods mentioned in the other chapters could be used for evening snacking. I use the tryptophan/niacinamide combination just described because it helps quiet the mind in preparation for sleep. For this reason, one can take

digestive enzymes

larger amounts near bedtime; 1500 mg would not be inappropriate.

There's another excellent way to handle after-dinner snacking, and that is to treat the gastrointestinal tract. Problems along the digestive tract are more common than once thought. Gas, irritable stomach, constipation, and diarrhea are extremely common. They signify the possibility of malabsorption of foods. It has been confirmed that both protein and carbohydrates may be incompletely digested before they are absorbed. This causes hypersensitivity reactions such as nervousness and hunger: the allergic syndrome.

Taking digestive enzymes can alleviate this problem in many people. If digestive enzymes are taken at supper, after-dinner cravings often disappear. I suggest three or four with dinner. After about a week, many patients report either a decline or a complete absence of cravings in the evening, and so long as the enzymes are continued, they don't return.

Many kinds of digestive enzymes are available at either health food stores or drugstores. Look for the combination of pancreatic enzymes and bile salts. If the tablet contains some betaine and lipotropics, it's even better.

MIDDLE-OF-THE-NIGHT CLOCK CRAVINGS

It's 3 A.M. and you're hungry

Middle-of-the-night cravings are a familiar plight. A person wakes in the middle of the night craving something, usually carbohydrates. He or she cannot go back to sleep without a snack. An occasional bout with the 3 A.M. munchies isn't too significant, but if it happens often it can lead to weight problems. There are a number of reasons why this occurs. It could be hypoglycemia, for the adrenal gland does shut down at about 3 A.M., and the blood sugar dips low enough to interrupt sleep. Anyone who has worked in a hospital will tell you how frequently the staff sees heart attacks at this time. Pregnant women seem to begin labor or deliver at around three in the morning, and emotional problems tend to peak at that gloomy hour. The coincidences are hard to ignore. All we can infer is that the body's chemistry can easily become imbalanced in those hours before dawn.

And there's one more explanation. Hunger can be due to allergic withdrawal symptoms that are severe enough to awaken the person and cause discomfort until a neutralizing dose of food is eaten. We have discussed food allergies in enough detail earlier, so you understand the mechanism.

The best way to solve this problem is to find a way to maintain sleep. Someone who stays asleep doesn't have to deal with the hunger cravings. Both of the ways I'm going to suggest work quite well, but they work for different reasons. I suggest patients try one and then the other, to see which is most satisfactory.

A small piece of chicken with salt or a salted hard-boiled egg has kept many of my patients asleep through the night. This method works so well in some cases that it carries over into the morning and prevents that early-morning hunger, which seems to strike those with predawn cravings.

Tryptophan at bedtime can also induce sleep that won't be interrupted by hunger. If this fails, the tryptophan can be enhanced by using 50 mg niacinamide along with it. I don't usually use B_6 at this time because it keeps some people awake or causes restlessness. Another reinforcer is calcium. I prescribe two 11 grain dolomite tablets with 1000 mg tryptophan and half a teaspoon baking soda in a glass of water. There are enough possible combinations to choose from that success is easily assured.

If you suspect that your problem is hypoglycemia, try two 200 mg tablets of GTF (glucose tolerance factor) chromium together with the protein and salt snack already mentioned.

CHAPTER TEN

Children and the Rest of the Family

Statistics have shown that women comprise the unlucky majority of victims of cravings. For that reason most of this book has been directed toward women rather than to men or to age groups such as children, teenagers, and the elderly. This chapter is devoted to the *rest of the family* and to preventing the development of permanent craving problems in the young.

CHILDREN

Can children have food craving? The answer is a definite yes. Ask any parent about his or her child's favorite food. How early can food allergies start? Children can be sensitized to foods before they are born. Studies have shown that overeating by the mother during pregnancy leads to allergies in the infant. This is especially true of carbohydrate foods like cookies, popcorn, and cereals.

The infant can also become allergic from breast feeding. If the infant is susceptible, it may fall prey to milk allergies. If a young child is overfed solid foods, the risk runs even higher. We all know the common desire on the part of parents to overnourish their young. But overfeeding a child during digestive upsets when the stomach is vulnerable, as sometimes happens, can encourage dangerous allergies.

Allergic symptoms are extremely common in infancy and early childhood. The highest incidence of food allergy develops during the first year of life, when eating is the infant's principal activity.

Parents are familiar with such allergic symptoms as colic, croup, diarrhea, and skin rashes. They are less familiar with identifying fevers, inability to toilet train, bed wetting, bronchitis, and colitis as unrecognized allergic symptoms. Most are aware that an allergy can cause behavior problems, but few, if any, know that it can manifest itself by a child's demand for a favorite food. In my experience, children with food allergies have a desire to eat constantly. The young allergic-addicted child never seems to get enough, especially sweets and bakery products.

Unfortunately, these cravings can also be seen in normal children who aren't at all allergic, causing considerable confusion for the parent. From time to time, when their metabolic rate increases, normal children eat more, too. The difference between allergy and normal growth needs may be subtle. However, the allergic overeater is more likely to be overweight, especially with a "potty" stomach. These children also prefer sweets, breads, and cheeses, whereas the hypermetabolic overeaters will often be satisfied with less fattening foods.

Woe to the young child whose parents do not alert themselves to the possibility of allergy and take action early. Unchecked overeating, especially of refined carbohydrates, bakery products, and milk products, can lead to serious health problems. Unchecked cravings in childhood can lead to irreversible obesity, diabetes, a bad self-image, poor schoolwork, laziness, and stubbornness akin to paranoia in adults.

You're never too young to have allergies, one of the symptoms of which is overeating. Once you recognize this possibility, you can take appropriate steps to block it.

Treat or trick

The junk food syndrome, a formidable threat to allergy resistance, starts with that first snack from Mom. Most mothers want their kids to have a treat, not always for beneficial reasons. Many times they bring home junk food more for their own sake. They want to have it around, either for their own occasional use or to enjoy it vicariously through their kids.

But then, like the drug buyer in a schoolyard, the youngsters get hooked on junk and begin to demand more. The first step to addiction can occur right at the outset with infant nutrition. With unwise selections come favorite-food problems, then outright food abuse, leading finally to addictive allergies.

Yeast infections in children

Yet another ever-present problem is the threat of yeast infections. Most newborn infants already have antibodies to molds. Some newborns develop yeast infection on the first day they enter the world. The mother's birth canal may be contaminated with large amounts of yeast, which enter the child's mouth as it passes through the birth canal. From then on, throughout the rest of its life, that child will be a host to the yeast. It may grow from the mouth downward into the gastrointestinal tract with the inevitable consequences: hunger and cravings.

Some doctors have raised the question of whether severe yeast infections in the mother could cause birth defects. There is no concrete evidence of this at present, but we do know that whatever immunity is functioning in the mother during pregnancy can be transferred to the child.

Candidiasis in children

By the sixth month of life, most babies show some positive reactions to skin tests for candidiasis. Infants are often given antibiotics for ear infections, throat infections, tonsillitis, bronchitis, or colds. Occasionally, these treated infants develop oral thrush, diaper rash, and diarrhea. Even if a child on antibiotics shows no symptoms of a yeast infection, it's probably a good idea to administer antifungal drugs if antibiotics are given.

Although most inner ear infections are caused by bacteria and not yeast, it is possible for both infections to be present. A thirteen-month-old patient of mine who had received antibiotics for an ear infection began to exhibit irritability, hyperactivity, fatigue, and bad behavior for several months afterwards. When I treated her for a *Monilia* infection, all of those symptoms disappeared within one day.

Parents of children who have chronic runny noses, restlessness, irritability, sleeplessness, or any other unhealthy symptoms should seriously consider the presence of candidiasis. If both the mother and the child are infected simultaneously, it's double trouble. Both may become irritable and fussy and may develop insomnia. The baby cries all the time, aggravating the mother's impatience. In extreme cases, this cycle may even lead to child abuse.

A six-month-old infant with Down's syndrome was brought to me for treatment. Prone to colds and chest infections, the patient was receiving antibiotics for an increasingly severe ear infection. The pediatrician was preparing to open the eardrums. However, I put the patient on a routine antifungal treatment, and within a week, all symptoms of the ear infection disappeared. In the following year none of the ear infection returned, and the infant had no infection problems other than a mild cough.

The message here is that the first symptoms of candidiasis are not hunger and cravings, but physical distress. If you as a parent don't recognize these developing symptoms, you are not only going to have a chronically sick child but one with an excessive appetite and weight problem.

It is a tragedy to see this type of situation become progressively worse. If there is no improvement, it sets a pattern that is difficult to reverse later in life. It may cause a child growing up to be overly concerned with his or her health, giving rise to a whiner, a complainer and, even worse, a dependent, helpless individual. These children become more inclined to manipulate their parents and use their illnesses as a weapon to get what they want.

If allergy symptoms occur, the family doctor may tell the

parent that the child will grow out of it. But this will not be the case if these symptoms are due to candidiasis.

If the *Candida* infection occurs during the child's first school years, a learning disability can develop. If this persists too long, it can set a future standard for the child's entire mood and attitude. Students with "C" and "D" grades have improved their grade point averages after being treated for candidiasis.

Any child who has a behavior or scholastic problem should be considered a possible victim of chronic fungus infection. Behavior problems often disappear when this infection is controlled. As a result, chronically hyperactive children with bad tempers or just plain mean personalities will finally begin to develop better manners along with improved schoolwork. Some kinds of behavior problems due to hyperactivity can be manifested in adults as depression, frustration, and bad temper—all the result of yeast byproducts affecting the nervous system.

Obesity in children

Excessive appetite provoked by allergy infections can affect body weight to an alarming degree. If severe enough, it can traumatize the body and often trigger a dramatic change in metabolism. The result: obesity.

In almost all such cases, intense cravings develop. If you have an overweight child with an irrepressible appetite, you can be sure there is a physical problem. If the child overeats when upset, don't deceive yourself into thinking it's a psychological problem.

Allergic cravings in children are very difficult problems to handle alone. The organizations and doctors in the last chapter should help you get started. You need to understand this problem fully if you are to cope with it.

TEENAGERS

To the parents of teenagers

Perfectly normal teenagers can drive parents to drink. Their obnoxious behavior is nothing new, all part of the process of growing up. But it's sometimes very difficult to control because teenagers today have greater mobility. At no other time in history have they been so able to go where or when they like. Teenagers are a strong consumer market subject to peer pressure from other teenagers. The junk food craze has become such a powerful influence that teenagers develop allergies as a result.

Given the fact that you cannot always control what your teenager eats, you still must be a guiding force over his or her diet. Offering them education about what junk food does to them can go a long way. You might even get some cooperation.

To the teenager

Most likely you know how junk food affects your weight, and you have probably suspected that it can affect your skin. I can assure you that acne and other skin conditions are made worse by junk foods. If you have a bad complexion, controlling your craving for junk food can help.

You might want to do better in school. Junk food, especially sugar, can give you hypoglycemia, a blood sugar problem that can affect your memory and your concentration. In turn, this can affect your grades. Cravings for foods that cause allergies can also disturb your concentration and even affect your memory. There are cases on record of teenagers who significantly raised their grade point average after they controlled their food allergies.

Finally, would you like to be less depressed, less moody, and feel more together? You've been around, so you know you have to give something to get something. Make good use of the simple ideas in this book and you can stop the junk food habit that is causing all those mood swings. For example, cut down on coffee and diet colas. They act in the same way as sugar. They destroy the delicate chemical balances that affect our moods. Our bodies were built to keep our moods on a steady keel. When we upset these balances, often everything seems to go wrong.

Candidiasis and teenagers

Poor judgment and reasoning abilities can be symptoms of candidiasis. When a girl or boy in the early teens suddenly switches from a happy, energetic good student to someone afflicted with confusion, mood changes, irritability, depression, and a decline in grade point average, the answer may be candidiasis. This abrupt mood shift may accompany signs of excessive hunger and radical weight changes.

There are cases of well-adjusted "A" students who suddenly seem unable to think or learn and become withdrawn and unable to communicate. As the concerned parents become frantic, the helplessness of the teenager intensifies until everything seems magnified out of proportion. It's an overwhelming burden that could change quickly if the causative factors were recognized.

The greatest misconception concerning these personality changes is that the cause is psychological. If you're considering consulting a child psychologist in such a case, it might be wise first to talk to an allergist or a clinical ecologist. If a teenager exhibits sudden personality changes at the same time he or she suddenly develops asthma, chronic headaches, or skin disease, especially after using an antibiotic, the cause might in fact be candidiasis. And in teenage girls, candidiasis often throws the menstrual cycle off balance and causes moodiness and emotionalism.

All this can be very confusing to the physician because the growing pains of adolescence are often attributed to emotional instability. It is not uncommon to see a great tide of emotions flowing in contrary directions as the teenager tries to adjust to life.

Depressed teenagers with thoughts of suicide should also

be considered for candidiasis evaluation. The suicide rate among teenagers is rising, and it is possible that a certain percentage of these victims could have been helped with candidiasis therapy.

Of course, you can't blame every teenage behavior problem on candidiasis. Much of it may indeed be psychological in origin. There are so many factors involved in the inappropriate behavior of teenagers that it is certainly not easy to predict what percentage of these problems can be attributed to yeast infection. You should always consider alternative possibilities, such as physiological factors. Even in the area of drug abuse, there have been reported cases of teenage drug addiction completely eliminated without any relapses by the treatment of yeast infection. Teenagers with the aforementioned symptoms often find relief with the proper treatment.

STEVE: AN ATTACK OF THE "FUNGUS"

Steve, a college student who had done well his first year, was suddenly bothered by what he thought was an asthma attack. Since he had had a long history of nasal allergy, his nasal polyps were promptly removed to help cure his wheezing. Then his grades began to deteriorate. He was treated for breathing difficulties and what appeared to be an allergy attack. Over the next year, his grades declined dramatically.

Fortunately, he was able to find an allergist who knew about clinical ecology. Although the patient's skin test showed nothing significant, the allergist suspected he did have a yeast infection because of his history of increased symptoms during weather changes.

Once *Candida* treatments were started, there was an immediate improvement. His fatigue and clouded thoughts disappeared, his irritability diminished, and most important, his grades improved considerably. The longer the treatment, the better his grades; his grade point average skyrocketed in his last semester. This improvement continued through graduate school. This case illustrates dramatically that even the impairment of brain function can be caused by yeast toxins.

GERRY: SWEETS AND DEPRESSION

At age 13, Gerry developed a bad case of acne. His family doctor prescribed the antibiotic tetracycline, but the acne improved only slightly. After six months, Gerry began to feel tired all the time, suffering nervous apprehension and nightmares. His schoolwork suffered; he spent less time with his friends and more time watching television because he was too fatigued to undertake anything more active. He ate sweets constantly and gained weight. High doses of vitamins could not revive him. His parents tried to persuade him to eat better foods, but away from home he gorged on junk foods. His depression worsened, and he started to miss school.

The family doctor put Gerry on a diet. His symptoms diminished and he lost weight, but soon his cravings overwhelmed him and he was eating sweets again. As a last resort, his parents turned him over to a psychologist. That, too, proved futile.

Finally Gerry found a doctor who started him on a treatment for yeast infection. He began to sleep better. He no longer craved sweets and junk food. Gradually, he lost weight. Better days came with mental improvement, and his depression lifted. It took two years of treatment before he was close to returning to normalcy.

Sudden weight gain

Sometimes a naturally thin teenager suddenly gains weight dramatically. If his or her resistance to disease also seems to be getting lower and frequent vaginal infections or stomach pains develop, this adolescent may be a victim of candidiasis. Teenage girls with delayed periods may also be on the victim list, even though emotional stress could also be the cause. The teenager may become constipated or may have diarrhea. Sometimes the only symptom is an increasing number of allergic responses. Constant dental problems also may be due to candidiasis.

Deadly snacks

The general assumption has been that snacks between meals not only discourage a proper regimen of regular meals, but are nutritionally harmful. The truth is not so clear-cut. It has been estimated that 25 to 35 percent of all food eaten daily by teenagers is in the form of between-meal snacks. While these foods are not all high-calorie, nutrition-poor foods, they consist for the most part of sugar. Consequently, large-scale consumption of snack foods has become a major problem.

Teenagers will seize any opportunities to eat away from home in snack-oriented establishments where they can gather socially and eat for the pure fun of it. Adolescents have the worst eating habits of all age groups because of their independence coupled with a lack of responsibility and maturity.

Teenagers often snack between meals two or three times a day. Their favorites are breakfast cereals, pies, cakes, milk, soft drinks, fruit, candy, potato chips, nuts, bread spreads, and apple sauce, to name a few. Eighty percent eat snacks after school and again after supper.

One of the most insidious problems is soft drinks and colas. Adolescents love them. Full of sugar, caffeine, phosphorus, and virtually nothing else, they can become highly addicting. Soft drink sales are doubling every two years, a tribute to their popularity.

Without a doubt, food is the major form of entertainment in this country today. Much of it is consumed for sheer pleasure rather than nutritional needs.

MEN

In men, yeast can find a home not only in the intestinal tract, but in the prostate gland. Women become emotionally volatile with *Candida* infection, whereas men react differently. Men are more susceptible to chronic tiredness or a bad disposition. Because men's emotions are not assumed to be cyclic like women's, the underlying problem is more easily overlooked. The family may assume that Dad's chronic complaining is just a male eccentricity setting in with age.

The symptoms of candidiasis in men are insidious. They may first notice difficulty in concentrating on their work. They may develop lapses of memory or a decrease in athletic performance. They may have more trouble keeping up with the demands of their jobs. Their sex drive may even diminish. These symptoms may slowly erode their self-confidence and adversely affect their accomplishments. On the physical side, men may develop intestinal symptoms, become chronic sufferers of allergies, or acquire an almost hypochondriac tendency toward infections. It is much easier to overlook problems like these in men than in women.

Men tend to drink alcohol or beer in response to this imbalance, rather than increasing food intake, including sweets. Alcohol and beer, a liquid form of starches, act like pure carbohydrates. Because the yeast allergy tends to thrive on carbohydrates, the result could be an addiction to alcohol or beer. Once again, the underlying condition must be treated to eliminate the problem.

ELDERLY PEOPLE

This group is the hardest of all to stereotype because we are dealing with a broad spectrum running from the cantankerous old fool to the wise elder. Golden agers are just as inclined as anyone to eat junk food, and they suffer more health problems from their indiscretions than anyone else. They are often just as rebellious and uncooperative as the teenager. Nevertheless, there isn't a treatment here they can't use profitably.

THE JUNK FOOD PHENOMENON

America is supposed to be the country of junk food addicts. However, in rural areas of Japan where there are no McDonald's or Jack-in-the-Box's many people die at an early age from the typical diet.

It's a junk food world

Medical studies in Japan can help us understand why environment and habit can overwhelm and overbalance bodily needs. In Japan, stroke is one of the most common causes of death, thanks in part to the high level of salt intake. Rice is a staple of nutrition, and large amounts of salt in the form of soy sauce are used as a condiment. In some areas very few people live past the age of 70 because large amounts of salt in the diet apparently lead to high blood pressure and stroke. Where potassium-rich seaweed is frequently eaten, on the other hand, there are many people over 70.

The point is that humans and animals adapt as best they can to their environment. They may not be conscious of an underlying malnutrition, so they have no motivation to migrate to an area better suited for health.

The body only demands more, in the form of an appetite or craving, when there is an *acute* deficiency. Long-term or *chronic* deficiencies don't have quite the same effect. (They don't change the appetite.) Despite our often indiscreet food intake (too much salt, too much oil, too much sugar, etc.), our bodies manage to make adjustments and compensate for us on a day-to-day basis. Hence we survive.

The level at which we function as we survive, however, can be adversely affected. Our level of accomplishments, our psychological needs, consciousness, concentration, and judgment-making process can all suffer if the body is not functioning up to par.

Despite the abundance of quality foods at our fingertips, many of us suffer from malnutrition because of our poor choice of diet. Our bodies cannot make the choices for us, so it's up to our brains to make the right decisions. We should not allow ourselves to become garbage disposals for junk food.

I've been all over the globe and found that today's world is indeed a junk food world. Big Mac and Jack-in-the-Box haven't yet taken over the planet, but each country has its native junk food. Despite starvation in Ethiopia, there are millions of Third World children busily gobbling up every treat they can get their hands on. Even in poverty-stricken countries, most natives have access to junk food. It's not just "America's problem."

Junk food gourmet style

Even high-class restaurants are guilty of offering so-called "healthy" dishes that are merely disguised junk food. It never ceases to amaze me that hamburger-stand food is condemned as junk food, whereas a fancy expensive restaurant is considered to be a place where one can "eat right."

I attended a gourmet cooking class at a very exclusive eating establishment in southern California. We were taught to prepare split-pea soup by first boiling a whole chicken, then removing it from the pot. To a gallon of greasy chicken base stock we added an equal amount of pure cream, a generous gob of butter, a cup of refined sugar, split-pea concentrate, a little ham, and some spices. Voila! The perfect appetizer—for a gallbladder attack! Ouch!

A four-star restaurant will serve the creamiest salad dressings, the richest sauces, buttery vegetables, ad nauseum. The calories are astronomically higher than found in your common drive-thru fast-food stand. These taste-enrichers are far more hazardous to your health than any greasy-spoon hamburger. After all, only the rich can afford gold-plated junk food.

The salt munchies

The universal craving for salty foods has reached epidemic proportions. Salt cravers rarely acknowledge that it's the salt they hanker for. They'd rather put the blame on the food itself, such as chips, cheese, ham, sauerkraut, peanuts, crackers, pretzels, potato chips, olives, pickles, and bacon. If you want to get a better idea of the high salt content of, say, regular supermarket cheese, try a taste comparison with a slice of unsalted cheese. The difference is astonishing. You may have a junk food habit that in actuality stems from a craving for salt, and not even know it.

Solutions for snackers

My prescription? Take one 500 to 1000 mg tablet of pantothenic acid at 10 A.M., one at 2 P.M., and one-half at 7 P.M. This seems to work well for adults and teenagers, but I wouldn't recommend it for children. Pantothenic acid may eliminate your need for a snack altogether or will at least reduce it to a smaller amount.

For candy and chocolate cravers, I would suggest two to four 11 grain tablets of dolomite and two to four 150 microgram (mcg) tablets of kelp whenever needed. If you suspect part of your problem is hypoglycemia, add a hard-boiled egg lightly salted to the dolomite and kelp.

Bakery products can be counteracted by four 150 mcg tablets of kelp every two hours during snack times. And a glass of spring water with ice and lime can provide a refreshing substitute for that diet cola without your having to feel deprived of your fix.

Snacking to kill boredom

One of the biggest reasons for snack craving is boredom. Many of my patients report, "I don't eat because I feel hungry—I eat because I'm bored." Boredom occurs more from lack of movement than lack of interest. The only true antidote is action. Listing interesting things to do on slips of paper and following through on them is one way to fight boredom. You can keep the slips in the cookie jar or refrigerator and pick one out whenever the urge to snack strikes.

Another way to handle this problem is to use a calming agent. An herb called passion flower works well as a relaxant, as does 100 mg niacinamide plus 25 mg vitamin B_6. In some cases, I have prescribed muscle relaxants to block overeating from boredom—and it worked.

For children aged 5 to 10 I would simply scale down the adult doses given above. For children under 5 who overeat, however, I would recommend 7½ grain alfalfa capsules. You can open the capsules and empty one into the child's food. Alternatively, you can combine the alfalfa with one teaspoonful of liquid calcium, which can be taken in a beverage. Most important, *don't* bring junk food into the house. If you're taking your children to the movie theater or some other repository of junk food, give them a sensible meal before leaving home. If they're not hungry, they are less likely to plead for snacks.

Healthy snack alternatives

Picking at food is an inevitable activity for you or your children. So if you're going to empty the kitchen of junk foods, find a reasonable substitute. Try stocking the refrigerator with bite-sized portions of apples, frozen bananas, cantaloupe, or melon balls. These fruits are low calorie and tasty if chilled. Ripe grapefruit wedges are quite sweet and delicious. Just use your imagination. Keep fruit or vegetable juice on hand to avoid urges for Coke, Kool-Aid, or other sugary beverages.

CHAPTER ELEVEN

Premenstrual Cravings

MARGE: TWO PEOPLE IN ONE

Marge B., a 38-year-old secretary, sat beside my desk sobbing hysterically; a minute or so later she was dramatically recomposed and in control. Then the tears began to flow again, as she futilely blotted her cheeks with an already soaked handkerchief. It was five days before her menstrual period and she was sinking rapidly into premenstrual depression. There were external reasons for her upset as well; she had just been fired from a good position, and her boyfriend had left her.

Marge lost her boyfriend and her job because of erratic aggressive behavior which occurred nearly two weeks out of every month. This time her symptoms had cost her more dearly than usual, but it wasn't the first time this had happened. Unless a change occurred, it wouldn't be the last time, because Marge had a history of broken romances and career changes.

Marge is basically a competent person, honest and reliable, but when her premenstrual symptoms begin, she changes into "evil personified"—sarcastic, hypercritical, insulting, intolerant, conniving, trouble-making. As soon as her period starts, out comes the "other Marge" again—compassionate, fun loving, and responsible.

Marge, fortunately, had a caring family who stood behind her, but even they had their limits. They sent her to three different therapists who counseled her and prescribed tranquilizers and antidepressants. She was dopey and unable to function at work, and worst of all, the medicines merely dulled rather than cured her symptoms. Medical consultations also were of little help. The pain pills and water pills prescribed did not change her dual personality.

Marge had one other symptom worth mentioning—premenstrual cravings for sugars and chocolate, and occasionally for alcohol. For days she fought with the cravings, never successfully. Although many women gain weight from these cravings, Marge was lucky. She didn't. But she did not entirely escape the side effects of too much sugar, for it caused her to suffer black depressions and hopelessness. She knew sugar was the catalyst, but she couldn't stop eating it.

I treated Marge for premenstrual syndrome (PMS) using progesterone, and her symptoms responded beautifully. Besides treating her medically for PMS, I sent her to a psychologist. On her first visit to the psychologist, even though she was premenstrual, her new control was so successful that she remained calm even as she related her long history of self-destructive behavior. Truly, Marge had a new control she never believed possible. Another happy result was that the new self-possession extended to her cravings. She stopped bingeing on sweets and chocolate each month. Not eating all that sugar also contributed to her self-discipline, for she was now freed of the blues that usually resulted.

What is PMS?

The average reader is probably aware of PMS. There are numerous articles appearing in women's magazines and a flood of new books that discuss the subject in detail. But women who are still a little unsure should take the test in the box.

Did you check off most of the items? If so, you probably

PMS CHECKLIST

Before Your Monthly Menstruation Do You: Check if yes

1. Seem to go crazy? ( )
2. Get depressed? ( )
3. Have difficulty smiling, lack a sense of humor? ( )
4. Get more tired, fatigued? ( )
5. Have increased hunger? ( )
6. Crave sweets? ( )
7. Feel mentally "off"? ( )
8. Have strong mood swings? ( )
9. Get irritable? ( )
10. Get waterlogged, gain weight? ( )
11. Have breast soreness? ( )
12. Get headaches? ( )
13. Become hypoglycemic (get weak if you don't eat)? ( )
14. Get acne, facial breakouts? ( )
15. Have more trouble with your allergies? ( )
16. Experience voice changes (hoarseness)? ( )
17. Have a bloated abdomen? ( )
18. Have painful joints? ( )
19. Get hay fever, runny nose? ( )
20. Lose sense of smell? ( )
21. Experience dizziness? ( )
22. Get bladder, urinary infections? ( )
23. Get boils, styes, herpes simplex (canker sores)? ( )
24. Have increased desire for alcohol? ( )

In addition, do you:

25. Have the same symptoms and problems during ovulation (midway between periods)? ( )
26. Have spasmodic symptoms or miss periods? ( )
27. Get colicky lower abdominal pains? ( )
28. Have painful intercourse at time of period? ( )

have premenstrual syndrome. "But wait," you say, "a mere written têst can't diagnose PMS. Aren't there laboratory tests that will give me a more concrete answer?" Actually there aren't, but in the last three to five years, women's groups have aroused public interest enough to create pressure on the scientific community. The fervor is now high enough to start more in-depth investigations into the problem.

PMS has always existed, but medical literature on the subject only goes back a scant 50 years. The symptoms of PMS seem endless: irrational behavior, anger, impatience, intolerance, hypersensitivity, moodiness, bloating, breast soreness, abdominal cramps, headaches, and so on. These symptoms begin at ovulation (middle of the monthly cycle) or later and continue until the onset of menstruation, and sometimes longer.

The University of Illinois Medical Center has identified the major sign of PMS to be a *total lack of self-control*. The sought-after control usually returns once the menstrual flow begins. In patients I have treated, symptoms occur just before the menstrual period, but PMS can actually show up any time of the month. Dr. David Rubinow of the National Institute of Mental Health has also reported that the so-called "premenstrual symptoms" may actually occur throughout a woman's cycle.

"It's all in your head"

I have treated a large number of patients for PMS, and one of the most common complaints I hear is "my family doctor says it's all in my head. He says there is no such thing as PMS." Family doctors who do take the patient seriously usually run several general health tests and perhaps a few hormone tests. If the results are normal, they tell the patient "I can't find anything wrong" and refer them to a shrink. Most women do not go. As I mentioned, there are no reliable tests for PMS, so a doctor can't make a definitive diagonsis. The patient is still on her own, confused and frustrated.

My experience is that many clinicians still believe that PMS is primarily a psychological disorder, while most research scientists believe it is not. They tend to believe that hormonal dysfunction is the cause.

Men, too, are often blind to what's happening. When patients are irritable, depressed, or cross before their periods, husbands and boyfriends may accuse them of using PMS as an excuse for bad behavior. Some men are so opinionated and closed-minded that nothing can breach their impenetrable wall, and empathy and understanding don't exist.

But even women sometimes turn a deaf ear to their own problems. Full of doubt and guilt about PMS, they oscillate between accepting it as a physical occurrence and scolding themselves for being so weak. After all, shouldn't they be able to exert some self-control?

One thing appears consistent: The more ''normal'' a woman's biochemistry, the less PMS she will have, and the more abnormal her biochemistry, the worse her symptoms will be. I have found over 50 percent of my patients with severe PMS also have other biochemical imbalances: excessive fears and phobias, mucocutaneous candidiasis, and strong allergic reactions to chemicals (and sometimes drug addictions).

What sets off PMS?

A number of situations seem to trigger PMS, including surgical procedures and taking birth control pills. Sometimes there is no identifiable cause.

Tubal ligation. A significantly large number of patients have complained to me that their PMS began directly after a tubal ligation. When I asked other doctors who treat PMS if they had received similar reports, their replies were positive. Although there are no studies to substantiate it, my observations make it worthy of consideration.

Birth control pills. Although contraceptive pills have been used to control PMS, it is also possible that they may unbalance the hormones enough to be a cause. Many of my patients say their symptoms first started while they were on the pill.

Hysterectomy. A number of patients have reported symptoms similar to PMS after surgical menopause. These symptoms did not exist prior to the surgery, but they afterwards began occurring on a cyclic schedule of one or two weeks once a month. These cases usually respond, I have found, extremely well to PMS treatment.

Dilation and curettage (D and C). The surgery known as D and C has also been reported to trigger PMS. It seems that any trauma to the uterus or ovaries may set off some change that results in a functional disease (a physiological imbalance).

No known cause. Mrs. P. came to me reporting PMS, which she had experienced for the preceding nine months. It had begun without apparent reason and had become progressively worse. I find that while more than half of my PMS patients can identify the trigger to their problem, a good number cannot.

Cravings and PMS

There are millions of women who crave foods only before their periods. The uncontrolled eating of chocolate, sugars, salt, and bakery products causes countless problems from weight increase to acne. So it is essential to find a resolution to their dilemma.

Since there is no *one* reason why women get PMS, it is obvious that we don't always know why associated cravings occur. Hypoglycemia has sometimes been blamed; those who subscribe to this theory recommend frequent small meals to keep the blood sugar more normal and the appetite down.

Readers of this book already know that such a regimen will not work. It may provide some control, but there's not a chance of it stopping an authentic chocolate mania.

It has also been suggested that a craver eat the foods she craves, but only a few bites. Realistically, if she had that kind of self-control, she could have stopped before the first bite. Let me give you examples of the willpower of PMS patients. I recently saw a woman who was in a reducing program at a major university. She was told to cook a chicken when she was premenstrual and to eat only a small portion of it if she got hungry. The first time her appetite was aroused, she ate the whole bird. I have talked to patients who have eaten several large cakes at one sitting when premenstrual. A box full of donuts or sweet rolls is a mere snack to a true carboholic. One or two bites and then stop? Forget it.

Tests for PMS

As I already said, there are currently no tests that conclusively say, "Mrs. Jones, you have PMS." That is not to say that there aren't tests to measure the level of hormones which control the menstrual cycles.

Prolactin is a hormone related to the monthly cycle. Research has linked it to PMS. If it's at a high level in your system, there are drugs you can take to lower it, but dealing with high levels isn't always the answer. I have seen a number of women who have had high prolactin levels lowered by the appropriate drug. They still had PMS. Prolactin may be linked to PMS, but changing the levels doesn't necessarily control cravings.

In the case of *thyroid hormones*, the theory is that a low thyroid level inhibits ovulation and causes unbalanced estrogen/progesterone ratios. This leads to PMS and cravings for chocolate and sweets. The treatment then would be to take thyroid pills. My experience is that thyroid medication either doesn't help at all or helps only minimally.

Follicle stimulating hormone (FSH) and *luteinizing hormone* (LH) are formed in the anterior pituitary gland. The brain uses these hormones to regulate estrogen/progesterone ratios during phases of the female cycle. When their action is not coordinated, the ratios become abnormal and PMS results. That's the theory, anyway. Unbalanced or not, these hormones don't help the doctor stop PMS or prevent premenstrual cravings.

An imbalance of *estrogen and progesterone levels* may be responsible for PMS. If the ratio is found to be abnormal, progesterone may be given by injection. Progesterone is very effective in relieving premenstrual cravings. There are, however, two problems related to this therapy. First, progesterone by injection must be given frequently, before each period, and these office visits create expense and nuisance for the patient; and, second, the oral progesterone tablets seldom work. I will discuss another form of progesterone later in this chapter. I have seldom seen supplementary estrogen decrease PMS. In most cases it only worsens the condition.

Maureen Dalton, M.D., has written an excellent book called *Once a Month* (Hunter House, Inc., 1979). In the book she describes sex hormone binding globulin (SHBG). She believes a low level of this hormone may indicate a diagnosis of premenstrual syndrome, although not many experts agree with her.

Progesterone and PMS

Progesterone is a hormone that controls the second half of a woman's monthly cycle. Some doctors have suggested that it sensitizes the body so that even small changes in blood sugar create a craving. In other words, progesterone in some ways *causes* the sugar cravings. As a further example of this, progesterone levels are high during pregnancy, a time when a woman's cravings may be much more intense.

I personally believe this theory to be incorrect. Many doctors give progesterone to patients with PMS; when they do, the cravings disappear within half an hour. In fact, considering the various methods used to control PMS cravings, I can't think of anything that is more certain to bring relief than progesterone.

As for the craving women have during pregnancy, there is abundant evidence pointing to mineral imbalances, not progesterone excess. Pica, the eating of dirt or other unusual materials, is not uncommon among expectant mothers. In one case, I saw a young woman with pica who would sometimes find herself overwhelmed by this desire. While walking along a city street one day, she became obsessed. She found a vacant lot between two houses and ate dirt by the handfuls. When she boarded a bus, her mouth and teeth were caked with dirt, which alarmed the other passengers and embarrassed the woman.

We have just indicated that excessive progesterone does not cause cravings, but we did not say that it plays no part. It does affect cravings, but the exact mechanism is not known. Possibly, PMS could be an endocrine allergy. A few doctors view this as a possibility, but medical literature on the subject is scarce. I was able to trace this concept as far back as 1954. When the estrogen/progesterone ratio is out of balance, there can be a relative deficiency of progesterone. This is quite probable, because the cravings disappear when we administer progesterone.

How progesterone relieves cravings

If you have only mild PMS symptoms, you probably won't need to employ this approach, so go directly to the next section on supplements. If your PMS cravings are moderate to severe, you might elect to try progesterone. It is a reasonably safe medication when properly used, but it must be taken under a doctor's supervision.

Dr. Maureen Dalton gives suppositories of progesterone which stop premenstrual symptoms, including cravings. Each one lasts for about four to six hours. In general, they are effective but cumbersome. For example, if you have a ten-day premenstrual problem and you take four to six suppositories a day, you will need 40 to 60 suppositories. That can be a nuisance as well as expensive. On the other hand, if you want to avoid PMS or premenstrual cravings, progesterone suppositories are worth considering. You'll have to get them from your physician or from one of the doctors belonging to the organizations listed in Chapter 16.

Supplements and PMS

Magnesium.   One of the most commonly suggested causes of PMS cravings is magnesium deficiency, and yet blood tests on PMS patients seldom reveal it. Dr. Jeffrey Bland in his book *Nutraerobics* says that magnesium is low in the blood cells of such patients. This was discovered by special lab tests. If red blood cells (RBCs) are studied instead of the blood serum, the magnesium deficiency becomes apparent.

One to three 100 mg magnesium tablets at the time a craving occurs can be effective, especially if reinforced by a 50 mg zinc tablet and a 50 mg B_6 tablet. One must be careful not to take amounts high enough to cause nervousness. Both B_6 and magnesium can cause hyperactivity.

Vitamin B_2 (Riboflavin). Another approach I have used with some success is to prescribe 25 mg vitamin B_2 tablets and suggest that a patient *chew* two or three when cravings occur. If it works, the cravings stop in 10 to 15 minutes. One important point: As soon as a patient regains control, I have her sequentially reduce the number of tablets until she can level off on the smallest amount that is effective, even if it's only half a tablet. Too much B_2 can unbalance the body as anything else can. As we know, when you unbalance the body, you increase cravings and risk creating additional problems as well.

Vitamin B_6. Vitamin B_6 appears to be the most overpromoted treatment for PMS today. Some women swear it helps, and I have no doubt it does in some of the milder cases. However, most of the patients I see for PMS say B_6 hasn't worked at all for them. It is also supposed to reduce tissue swelling (edema), but it frequently doesn't. By itself, it can be mildly effective or disappointing, and it certainly doesn't help cravings. On the other hand, it is very helpful as an assistant to other vitamins.

Supplement Combinations. You can use any of the combinations of supplements listed in the book, but here is one I have prescribed with some success. I have a patient take three 300 mg calcium lactate tablets along with one Complex F and a 50 mg niacinamide 10 mg B_6 tablet, from Standard Process Labs, when the cravings begin and each time they return, until control is stabilized. Regular niacinamide 50 mg tablets can be used in place of Standard Process niacinamide B_6, and three linseed oil capsules can be used instead of Complex F. Linseed oil capsules are all the same strength. For long-term control use one 400 unit vitamin E capsule, 400 mcg of selenium, and three evening primrose capsules daily for three months as a test. Continue indefinitely if it works.

General measures to prevent PMS cravings

As you know, if you can prevent PMS, you can stop cravings. There are many good books that provide helpful suggestions. In addition you can:

Get the man in your life on your side. If he isn't working for you, he may be working against you. There are plenty of inexpensive paperback books on PMS for him to read. If he refuses to do so, go through the book yourself, underline the important parts, and read them to him. In other words, you must educate him even if it takes time. If he is already well informed, ask him not to tempt you with sweets—especially when you are premenstrual. If he helps you resist these things, you will have less to fight.

Get sugar out of your diet. Cutting down on carbohydrates during the premenstrual period greatly helps decrease PMS. That means no sugar or sugary items. Eliminate fruits or restrict yourself to one daily; apples or cantaloupes are best. NO FRUIT JUICES: A common mistake is to think that concentrated fruit juice is healthful. It contains nutrients, but it also floods sugar into the body. Like refined sugar, these fruit sugars cause more water retention than salt.

Avoid caffeine, coffee, tea, colas, and chocolate. All of these rob the body of water soluble vitamins through diuresis. In addition, these items may cause hypoglycemia. There is absolutely no doubt that caffeine intensifies PMS.

Avoid alcoholic beverages. Alcohol is essentially pure sugar, and behaves like sugar in the body. It causes the same problems as sugar, and often more intensely.

Why are we telling you not to eat sugar or drink alcohol after we just told you how to block cravings? Because even if you block *cravings* for sweets or salt and thereby reduce your intake, you should also avoid eating problem foods through habit or in social situations. The idea is to not eat these foods *at all* when you are premenstrual, whether you crave them or not.

Exercise regularly. A number of patients have reported relief of premenstrual symptoms by embarking on an intensive exercise program during the last two weeks of each cycle. That means three to five one-hour sessions each week. Even if you don't get total relief, you will benefit from a regular exercise program.

Use evening primrose oil. This oil is the "Queen of the Supplements." It contains essential fatty acids that help restore balance to the body. Take four to six capsules daily for 14 days before each period and one to three capsules daily at other times of the month. The effects are usually not felt initially, but after three to four months, you should realize the full effect. If it works for you, there is a definite reduction in PMS and cravings.

Cravings: Hormones and the yeast connection

Attacking premenstrual cravings directly is perfectly proper, but one must not forget that PMS may be a disease by itself or it may be the symptom of another, more serious illness. Let's use yeast infection as our example.

How do yeasts cause hormone imbalances that can lead to PMS and cravings? The process has to do with the production of toxins that can block hormone action. The female sex hormones originate mostly in the ovaries. When released, they affect many organs of the body, including the skin and the brain, as well as the uterus. They cause the lining of the uterus to build up and then slough off in a cyclic manner, thus producing menstruation. Many nonsexual organs and tissues of the body are dependent upon female hormones for their proper functioning, and if they are not in proper balance, or if these tissues are not themselves receptive owing to blocked receptor sites, numerous symptoms will result.

How can we tell whether we are producing enough hormones or if these hormones are properly affecting the receptors on the cells? A doctor can check vaginal tissues. An unstimulated appearance indicates a lack of estrogen; if the blood estrogen levels are then found to be normal, we can see a discrepancy. The mucous membranes are not being stimulated even though there are adequate amounts of hormones in the blood. One of the processes that lead to this impairment is yeast infection.

In these cases, it does no good to prescribe hormones, because tissues cannot respond to them. The problem is not insufficient hormones; it is too little response to the hormones at the tissue level. In fact, the hormone treatment may not only fail but may cause further problems. It may have a domino effect on other endocrine glands of the body such as the thyroid or the adrenal glands. Most important, it may have some adverse effect on the pituitary gland. It makes a lot of sense to treat the *Candida* infection, if it is the cause of the blockage, before administering hormones. In many cases, treating the *Candida* infection alone is enough to cause the tissues to respond to the already adequate female hormones, and thus no hormone treatment will be necessary.

The point to be made here is that candidiasis and other fungal diseases can contribute to premenstrual symptoms and premenstrual cravings. I have just described to you how one fungus, *Candida albicans*, unbalances the body. If your cravings are the result of this more serious disease, that problem must be eliminated if you expect any long-term control of your cravings and significant relief from PMS.

CHAPTER TWELVE

Bulimia and Anorexia Nervosa

Do you have uncontrollable urges to eat huge amounts of foods in a short time? Do you get so upset from overeating that you *make* yourself vomit? Is each episode of bingeing and purging followed by feelings of guilt, remorse, and self-contempt? Do you use laxatives often to force the food out of your body? Do you have a terrible fear of fatness? If so, you are bulimic.

BULIMIA

A study by the University of Minnesota (Mitchell, 1981) found that bulimics binge an average of 14 hours a week. In the group studied, some patients consumed as much as 50,000 calories a day. That's equivalent to over 33 large pepperoni pizzas, or 350 Twinkies, or 100 banana splits, or 310 bags of corn chips, or 80 Burger King Whoppers, or 500 slices of American cheese. An old joke is don't eat anything you can't lift. Thirty-three large pizzas would seem hard to lift, let alone eat, yet this disease compels its victims to eat as much as fourteen pounds of food in one sustained binge within the time frame of a single day.

Victims are generally females who begin this unfortunate

pattern in their late teens. Shame and embarrassment cause them to become secretive. They often ingest food as if it were a liquid, barely chewing it. Sweet or starchy foods are most preferred.

Even though bulimic patients promise themselves never to overeat again, they are rarely able to change their behavior. Between binges, they often attempt to diet or abstain from food altogether, but normal eating patterns are almost never achieved. Preoccupied with food, weight control, and dieting, bulimic patients often refuse to eat with other people.

These individuals contend with sudden and powerful urges to overeat; they live in constant fear of not being able to stop eating, even though most of them are of average weight or even slightly thin. Some of the patients are bulimic during one period and anorexic at another, with behavior swings not unlike manic depressives. (Anorexia nervosa is discussed later in this chapter.) It is not unusual for there to be associated physical problems such as menstrual irregularities, headaches, stomach pains, and dizziness. It has also been noted that many of these patients have compulsive personalities; a few even border on psychosis.

Because bulimia is a "secret" disease and not readily observed by friends and family, it's difficult to gather statistics, but reports indicate that the phenomenon is far from rare. Like most forms of illness, this disease varies greatly in severity. Episodes can be mild and infrequent, or they may consume a patient's life.

Who should treat bulimia?

Professionals in a number of fields have claimed expertise in treating bulimic patients. Everyone from psychoanalysts to neurologists has taken a crack at it, with each group claiming to have the right answers.

Some research studies show binge eating to be due to neurological malfunction, possibly even to a form of epilepsy. Results of brain studies (electroencephalograms, or EEGs) are found to be abnormal in a certain percentage of cases, indicating that neurological factors do indeed play a role in some cases of compulsive eating. There's a possibility that some night eating may be neurologically based and may be related to bulimia in some way.

The anxiety factor

Many so-called normal people will binge during times of stress but will not carry on to the point of purging the food. Why are some people motivated to induce vomiting and others not? Researchers tell us that purging, as well as overeating, relieves anxiety.

It has been found that bulimic eating binges are primarily triggered by emotional upsets. These crises catapult the binger into high levels of depression and anxiety, which results in a feeling of being out of control. But instead of taking appropriate action to relieve the stress and solve the problem, bulimics stuff themselves with food in a wild frenzy, ending the orgy with guilt and fear.

Frozen with fear

We all know that some people overreact to situations that would merely annoy others. Bulimics may have an exaggeration of the normal response to everyday stress.

Most people can at some point be traumatized so severely that they feel totally out of control, and this produces the sensation of helplessness. Let me give you an example of a normal reaction to severe trauma. In one recent airline accident, the main cabin was not immediately destroyed. Most of the passengers were still alive and strapped in their seats. Many remained motionless, but a few unbuckled and fled to safety. A minute or so later, the cabin exploded in flames and those who stayed helplessly in their seats perished. Apparently these passengers were in such a state of shock that they were unable to take action. They were rendered helpless and incapable of even attempting to control the situation. So profound was their shock they could not recognize and take advantage of the minute or so of control within their grasp. Those 90 seconds of paralysis cost them their lives.

addictive substance defined as relieving
anxiety or depression

Panic and addictive behavior

Panic can cause a person to become too disorganized to deal with a problem; this feeling creates an urge to do something "crazy" or unwise. We call that being maladaptive. When you should be figuring a way to solve the problem, you instead become obsessed with relieving anxiety. Most of us are aware of the role this pattern plays in alcoholism and drug addiction. These substances remove the pain of anxiety, but not the problems.

Part of the definition of an addictive substance is that it relieves anxiety or depression. In the same vein, one may become addicted to behavior that relieves these conditions; this is defined as compulsive behavior.

Consumatory behavior

Bulimics must deal with a double load of anxiety. Whatever the intrinsic problem, they must also cope with the additional anxiety of overeating. Instead of relieving the first level of anxiety, food becomes a source for a secondary level of stress. This second level occurs when self-esteem is threatened by potential weight gain. Patients often consume a pound or more of food at one sitting. They may binge this way a dozen times a week, lending credence to their fears.

If either fight or flight is unavailable or is ineffective as a means of stopping anxiety, then consumatory behavior will often occur. Fear levels continue to rise if uncertainty persists, and one loses a grip on control. In a last-ditch stand to exert control in at least some small area, consumatory behavior results. In a crisis, we can always spend money on something pleasurable to consume. (When the going gets tough, the tough go shopping.) Sunday is mall day. Spending money is a major American entertainment. Sensual gratification is another. Many of our current forms of sexual pleasure are designed to prove our worth and desirability. But oral gratification has always been the first line of defense against anxiety. It is the easiest consumatory behavior to indulge in and a first-class way to get rid of anxiety.

Another look at anxiety:
The NE factor

Let's go back again to the crash of the airliner. Why didn't more of the passengers attempt to escape? Research has shown that the neurotransmitter norepinephrine, also called noradrenaline, is a factor in the will to live. In other words, NE plays a major role in emotional control. In some individuals, the supply of norepinephrine (NE) is quickly exhausted. When that happens, the person loses the desire to escape. This loss of will combined with a low energy level makes effective action difficult.

J. M. Weiss (1976) has shown that rats who are able to maintain control of a situation during electroshock have increased levels of NE in their brains. On the other hand, rats who are not able to control a shock situation show a decreased supply of NE.

I recently watched a neighborhood cat who had caught a field mouse and was playing with it. The mouse would try to escape. The cat would let it get a few feet away but then would quickly recover it before escape was complete. After this happened a number of times, the mouse gave up and abandoned all efforts. Even after the cat was taken away and could no longer endanger the mouse, it did not attempt to escape. It had resigned itself to death. After almost ten minutes of sitting alone in the center of the lawn, it finally recovered enough to begin to move gingerly away from the place of danger.

Research has shown that as soon as normal rats are presented with a way of regaining control of a situation, they immediately lose their sense of helplessness and organize a plan of action.

Researchers who have put rats in ice water for six minutes have noted a significant decrease in NE. When tested by shock 30 minutes later, the animals acted helpless and did not seek to escape. When a chemical was used to destroy NE in the brain, this too produced a failure to act.

In humans, low levels of NE may explain the feelings of helplessness experienced by some people. Many times the paralysis is not complete; instead of not acting at all, they turn to inappropriate substitute behavior. They act, but not in a way that will solve the problem. Norepinephrine decrease is not the full explanation for helplessness, though. There are other factors involved, but NE is part of the puzzle of self-defeating behavior. Readers who want to change such behavior should consider this information.

The basic message here is that if the anxiety that triggers cravings is physical, then we can rather easily contrive physical methods to block the experience. We will discuss this point again later in the chapter.

Thin skin

It has been suggested that bulimics suffer from low self-esteem. If that's true, we can assume that they have hypersensitive feelings. Excessive need for validation and affection indicates a need for constant approval. Of course, we all depend on others for positive feedback to some extent. When we are deprived of approval, we can easily become vulnerable.

If a person has a shaky ego, outside influences and opinions can be devastating. Greater than normal dependency on others for pleasure and happiness can produce fears whenever approval isn't forthcoming. Susceptible individuals have their antennae so fine-tuned that even unintentional slights can cause them to overreact. Because anger and self-pity often accompany hurt feelings, it's frequently necessary to keep one's feelings private so they will not be exposed to possible ridicule. Suppressed feelings, especially anger, can lead to addictive behavior.

Anger and self-abuse

Underneath the hurt is disguised anger—anger that one does not want to recognize, especially if it produces feelings of guilt. The bulimics I have seen have generally been "nice people" with low self-esteem. They are not easily provoked to anger. One of the reasons for hiding anger is that excessive fear sometimes suppresses it. Anger itself is a definitive way to control circumstances; if you deny that anger and bury it, you lose control over situations. This loss of control can lead to still more anxiety. Fear and anger are the two basic emotions used to combat problems—if someone has learned not to be angry, then he or she will respond by being afraid. Fear is unpleasant, so the person must then find a way to dissipate it. That way sometimes involves self-abuse, one form of which is bulimia.

Guilt

Guilt is produced by an act of wrongdoing, a delinquency. It's a panicky feeling of having taken a disapproved action —the feeling you get when a police officer pulls you over for a traffic violation. If you desire a psychological explanation, you could say that this type of fear is first experienced in the stomach, hence the term "gut-level." If you clean the stomach by vomiting, you can vomit out the fear as well.

Guilt is the immediate cause of purging, but the underlying problem is fear: fear of being fat, fear of being found out, and a general pervasive fear. All of these must be dealt with in therapy.

ANOREXIA NERVOSA

Anorexia nervosa is a disease that's been recognized for over a hundred years. Usually, the patient refuses to eat and is obsessed with being fat. Most all of the cases involve females from the United States and Europe. Earlier psychologists believed that anorexia was a form of hysteria, causing an individual to have an altered body image. Like bulimics, anorexics are usually young. Unlike bulimics, they are usually seriously underweight. Like bulimics, anorexics may induce vomiting or overuse laxatives. Many anorexics hide depression more effectively than bulimics. In both groups, amenorrhea (failure to menstruate) seems to suggest a hormonal relationship, but tests show no glandular abnormalities. The loss of menstruation is seen in bulimics and occurs in anorexics *before* they stop eating. If they later start to eat normally, the condition may continue, again suggesting a glandular problem.

Many of the symptoms of anorexia nervosa have been produced in patients by giving them high levels of estrogen. Animal studies have also shown anorexic symptoms after high levels of estrogen are given. The feeling of being bloated or overweight has also been described by patients with naturally high estrogen levels. It is interesting to note that this disease usually begins around puberty, when hormones are changing and estrogen levels are rising. Menopausal women, whose estrogen levels are low, do not seem susceptible.

In the *Journal of Psychology 1975* (Volume 3, 1975), researcher J. K. Young suggests that anorexia nervosa may be caused by estrogen overexciting a central area of the brain called the hypothalamus. It is a very powerful area. When the hypothalamus is overexcited, the condition can be fatal, which may explain why 15 percent of anorexics die of their disease.

Bulimia and anorexia nervosa: Is there a relationship?

Most researchers believe that these two diseases are related in some way, but at the moment, more concrete data are needed. The symptoms of the two groups seem to overlap: People in both categories are obsessed with thoughts about food. Both are diet conscious to the extreme and constantly worry about their weight. Both groups have an extreme desire to overcompensate as a safety factor to avoid being fat; they also have an extreme fear of losing control.

In bulimics, the binges are uncontrollable experiences that resemble some aspects of an epileptic seizure. Sometimes the bingers even feel detached from the experience. It has been said that such excessive behavior could only occur in a person with an illness.

No middle ground

Anorexics sometimes become bulimic. That is, they jump back and forth between the two extremes of bingeing and refusal to eat. Victims cannot seem to hit the middle ground; rather they seem to have separate states of mind, without ever stabilizing at a normal state. The bingeing is often described as a trance-like condition in which actions are out of the individual's control.

Both states of mind are rigid and not susceptible to change. There is no way to talk these patients out of the problem. Reason is useless. Direct attempts to change them causes additional insecurity, which leads to more self-abusive behavior. Then the vicious cycle begins again. They cannot establish a "normal state of mind" because they cannot achieve freedom from anxiety. These extreme states of mind have at times been described as "subpersonalities." Patients sometimes call it "the monster" or "devil" within. Much like the alcoholic, the patient may be unaware of the problem caused by the "other self."

If the problem is, in fact, a mental state, doesn't that prove the diseases are psychological rather than physiological in origin? Not necessarily. Mental states can be altered by physical factors. For example, one researcher found that when a single mineral, manganese, was removed from the diet of female rats, they lost all of their maternal instincts. The brain signals for maternal behavior were blocked. When the mineral was replaced in the diet, the maternal instinct returned. All of us may be "split personalities" to some minor extent. In the classical definition, as with true "multiples," one personality may not know the other exists, or knowing, may be helpless to control it.

It's been suggested that what keeps people bouncing between two extreme states is fear. They fear relaxing enough to assume normal equilibrium. Rather, fear becomes a part of both states of mind—the personality flip-flopping between them. The patient has the sense that a catastrophe will ensue if he or she doesn't stay in a particular state, but then the other personality eventually takes over.

Some of our compulsive behaviors such as smoking, eating, and alcohol abuse may be representative of this phenomenon. We develop different states of mind toward these behaviors, and they become so separate from the rest of us that we lose control over them. This is a simplistic explanation, but it has been used by the British therapist J. Hevesi, who claims to have an 80 percent cure rate with anorexics.

use zinc & B6 together

Is there a cure?

Most bulimics know they have problems and want help. They seem to respond much better to group or individual therapy than anorexics do, indicating that a less severe physiological disturbance is more easily treated. Patients often improve, at least temporarily, when in group therapy, in response to the support and security they receive. A combined approach of psychotherapy, nutritional supplements, and perhaps even drugs can help many bulimics. According to recent studies in both bulimia and anorexia nervosa, there may be an imbalance of zinc metabolism or some metabolic process related to it. Why does a zinc imbalance seem likely? One of the most important effects created by a zinc deficiency is loss of appetite, a major symptom of anorexia. When zinc is prescribed, there is a tremendous increase in appetite. If our zinc metabolism sputters on and off, we might see a gain and loss of appetite. Another interesting bit of information about zinc-disturbed individuals is that there is a dramatic reduction of motility (movement) of the gastrointestinal tract. This could create fullness and discomfort from overeating. Bulimics often say they experience severe bloating and pain after a binge.

Many anorexics report that food tastes unappetizing (another symptom caused by lack of zinc). A relative zinc deficiency may cause emotionalism. It is also important to note that this condition can lead to either anorexia or to pica, the eating of strange and unusual materials. Finally, zinc plays a role in insulin metabolism, which may have a relationship to hypoglycemia (another cause for overeating). No doubt there are many interesting connections between zinc and bulimia; the answer isn't simple, but zinc may play a role in the overall mechanism. Bulimia or anorexia nervosa often begins after a stringent diet, and we know that improper diets can cause zinc deficiencies, thus provoking the start of a vicious cycle.

If you are bulimic, you should be taking 50 mg of zinc three times daily. The purpose is not necessarily to block the cravings but rather to treat the underlying causes. In addition to zinc, it would be wise to take 100 mg of vitamin B_6—also three times daily. The two work better when used together. It would also be wise to take a strong multivitamin-mineral tablet at least once a day.

When a craving attack occurs, try two 400 mg phenylalanine tablets and 100 mg of niacinamide. Phenylalanine is an amino acid that is used by the body to manufacture norepinephrine and dopamine. These two substances prevent depression and decrease the appetite.

The precise dosage will be entirely up to you. Start with one tablet before each binge, and slowly build it up. Be aware that phenylalanine is a stimulant and may cause nervousness—so use it with caution. Note that the artificial sweetener Nutrasweet contains this chemical.

Phenylalanine can be made more effective by adding vitamin C crystals. Use one teaspoonful (4000 mg) immediately, along with 50 mg of B_6 and one 400 mg tablet of phenylalanine. You will have to keep these ingredients handy for immediate use so that a binge doesn't take you by surprise. A few minutes' delay, and panic will overpower your good intentions. Another ingredient that would complement this formula well is niacinamide. Start with 100 mg. Much more can be used in combination with the other formula.

Perhaps one of the best supplements for bulimia is L-glutamine, an amino acid that indirectly helps calm anxiety. I use four to six 500 mg L-glutamine tablets with two 200 microgram GTF (glucose tolerance factor) chromium tablets every three hours for one week. Then I lower the dosage frequency to three times daily, increasing it again if there are increased stressors or triggers to new craving attacks. Bulimics should also be using 400 mg of vitamin E, 400 micrograms of selenium, and either evening primrose oil, linseed oil, or cod liver oil—three capsules daily.

Bulimia is a serious disease and should not be taken lightly. It may very well be a form of epilepsy in some people, while in others it may indicate a hormone imbalance or some peculiar form of zinc deficiency. In any case, *you should not attempt to treat it without professional help.* Psychologists, psychiatrists, neurologists, and internists all offer treatment. If you think you suffer from it, seek advice immediately, because bulimia and anorexia nervosa can lead to even more serious illnesses and sometimes death. Don't delay. There is much that can be done for you.

PART FIVE

Additional Approaches

CHAPTER THIRTEEN

The Psychological Approach to Cravings

Everyone seems to admire people with willpower—those who have the foresight and will to give up certain bad habits. Their self-control will pave the way toward mastering their future. Strong people can endure painful deprivation to achieve their goals. A struggling college student will labor away year after year, isolated in poverty, for that coveted college degree. People with willpower control their environment instead of letting the environment control them. To many of us, willpower is a mystical force. To others it's simply a behavioral process by which one assumes responsibility for one's own welfare.

Psychologists, supposedly, have the professional insight to understand what skills are necessary to develop willpower. Unfortunately, most of them differ radically on what those skills are.

Willpower: To eat or not to eat

There is a widely held view that cravers and obese individuals seriously lack willpower. Their intense need for immediate gratification is so great that they forget the consequences of their actions (obesity, hypoglycemia, allergy, diabetes, hypertension). Overeaters overrespond to the sensations created by foods, until the pleasure of eating becomes an all-consuming obsession.

People with this attitude somehow overlook the fact that for the overeater, the consequences of *not* overeating are more unpleasant than they are for the so-called restrained eater. The overeater's so-called overresponse is actually caused by withdrawal symptoms that the "restrained eater" does not feel. Rather than seeking pleasure, the overeater is avoiding the agony of these withdrawal symptoms.

Once patients have been desensitized to an addictive food, they cease to overrespond to food cues. The food not only becomes less appealing to them, it becomes less gratifying in taste and texture and loses its "favorite food" status. It becomes just another food.

The current psychological view of an overeater's need for immediate gratification without any regard for the later consequences is a short-sighted one. It should be expanded to include the painful consequences of *not* overeating, which can be more overwhelming than any fear of future ill effects. Anyone stranded in the wilderness or lost at sea without food or water for weeks will feel "good," if not ecstatic with pleasure, after that first sip of water and a hot meal. Deprivation is so painful that relief from extreme hunger enhances taste and encourages one to overeat.

Willpower is easily defined in two simple words, "will" and "power." Will refers to the mind. Willpower equals mental energy. When you have energy you can have willpower. When you don't have energy, obviously you don't have willpower. Willpower to eat or not to eat depends on energy levels which come and go and cannot always be relied upon. It also depends, to a large degree, on our internal conversations with ourselves. We converse with ourselves constantly. The logical thing to do, it would seem, is to create new self-conversations if the old ones aren't working. If you talk to yourself differently, the argument goes, you will *act* differently.

The trouble is that this simply doesn't work with overresponsiveness to food. Thoughts can encourage feelings, but more often feelings determine thoughts. Withdrawal symptoms create such powerful feelings (feelings are more powerful than thoughts) that self-conversations tend to reverse themselves toward justifying the immediate relief of unpleasant feelings instead of blocking cravings.

Willpower can work, however, if you plan ahead and set up circumstances to protect yourself from temptation. It must be done when you are in a reasonable frame of mind, unbuffeted by overreactive emotions; once temptation starts to fire up these emotions, willpower may redirect itself toward what you want, not what you need. Nor does your body think in terms of the future. It only knows what it needs now. If your body cries out in pain because of a metabolism disturbed by withdrawal symptoms, only your mind will be able to understand the dangers your present behavior will create in the future. Otherwise, the body's immediate needs will force the mind into submission.

Appetite: Psychological or physical?

Most psychologists link excessive appetite to the expression of obsessive-compulsive rituals, acting-out behavior, or as a defensive mechanism to control tension. Cravings, in particular, are often attributed to hidden motives and meanings within the subconscious. The average psychologist therefore believes he or she can alter such cravings with psychological tools: psychoanalysis, psychotherapy, group therapy, hypnosis, or a dozen other professional techniques. Appetite and cravings are regarded as a learned behavior. The psychologist therefore believes that they can be remolded by conscious effort.

Veterinarians and scientists who experiment on animals, however, have a different perspective. Presumably, the food choices of animals are free of psychological motives. Laboratory animals do not always make the right selection. For example, if rats deficient in vitamins B_1 and B_6 are offered a choice of foods, some containing these vitamins, some not, they do not invariably select the right food. Of course, such foods are in themselves unnatural. Lab animals with sodium deficiency, on the other hand, do seek out salt. Salt does occur in isolation in nature.

Many studies show that pastured farm animals and animals in the wild are quite precise in their selection of needed foods. If laboratory rats under controlled experimental conditions fail to confirm these observations, the problem may be those same conditions. *The Chemical Senses and Nutrition*, Owen Maller (1967), suggests that domestication may have altered the rats' regulatory mechanisms. In addition, if a rat has only two or three choices, the experimenter has not really duplicated the unlimited choices found in its natural habitat.

Lastly, there is the paradoxical natural behavior in which harmful foods are sought or helpful ones ignored. For example, children with phenylketonuria or galactosemia will eat foods rich in phenylalanine or galactose even though these very substances cause severe illness. It is often difficult to get these patients to quell their desire for these foods. In other words, they crave the foods that harm them the most. These two diseases are not allergy addictions. The paradoxical behavior must be related to some totally different biochemical mechanism. So too may be the paradox of alcoholics who seem disinterested in essential nutrients necessary to help them metabolize out the alcohol and restore health. Yet there are also experiments that show that adults and children tend to select a good diet when there is a wide variety of foods available.

It seems clear that, at the least, physiology *and* psychology are at work here. But despite all this confusion and contradiction, the majority of psychologists still cling to the old theory that "it's all in your head." Fortunately, attitudes are changing. A small but growing coalition of professionals now argues that cravings and appetite may instead be the result of *biochemical* causes.

Weaknesses in the psychological approach

Psychological applications abound in our society. More and more people go to therapists now, not always with successful results. Psychological studies delve into every facet of life, and there are countless books, articles, talk shows, and news specials on psychological themes. We all know that psychology plays a major role in our lives. The real question is, what has all this done for us? And have the psychologists ever really proved themselves?

It's clear that the interaction between thoughts and emotions can quickly be physically expressed. If you get upset you may start to tremble, perspire, or blush; when deeply touched, you may shed tears. Extreme fear can provoke nausea, vomiting, even uncontrolled urination or defecation. In a confrontation with danger, our adrenal glands release adrenaline (epinephrine) to make us more mentally alert and able to cope with the situation. Our heartbeat quickens, raising our blood pressure to ensure that our brain has plenty of oxygen. These normal reactions are not consciously planned; they are physiological reactions.

Regrettably, the mind and body are not always perfectly coordinated. When emotional tensions arise, *abnormal* functions occasionally occur—exaggerations of a normal response to stress such as constipation. These symptoms are psychosomatic; that is, our mind is causing our body to change.

Some Eastern philosophies are predicated on the theory that there is little separation between mind and body because the cells of the body's tissues are thought to have their own intelligence and memory system. In Western science everything is broken down into the simplest possible categories; hence, doctors tend to overspecialize. Psychologists and psychiatrists explain psychosomatic symptoms only from their specialized, and often limited, point of view. The whole person is not always considered.

Unfortunately, if a specialist overemphasizes the psychological approach, physical causes may be totally ruled out to the detriment of the patient. The patient is labeled "psychoneurotic," which often eliminates a search for a physical cause of mental symptoms. This label often embarrasses the patient, who is left feeling the symptoms are his or her "fault." Once a diagnosis of psychoneurosis has been made, doctors tend to take a patient's physical symptoms less seriously.

Medical doctors claim that they are not prejudiced by a

psychological diagnosis. Nevertheless it does influence the physician's thinking and sometimes stigmatizes the patient. A psychiatric diagnosis also influences other people's reaction to the patient.

Overlooking physical causes

If the problem is an overlooked yeast infection or a food allergy, psychiatric treatment could continue for years with little change in the patient's symptoms or ability to function. As a result, the patient's sense of guilt and inadequacy will deepen with time. Patients begin to feel that they are using symptoms to avoid coping with the problems of life.

Some psychologists and psychiatrists may realize that if things are not improving with psychological treatment, some physical pathology may have been overlooked. Most, however, will assume they simply have not delved deep enough into the problem. They may decide to change their approach but will persist in seeking out mental causes for the patient's depression, anxiety, intellectual impairment, and the like. The consequence of such prolonged misinterpretation may cause neurosis in the patient who had none before.

Overselling psychology

Introspection is the most oversold commodity in our society. We dwell endlessly on our stress, anxiety, emotional insecurity, and lack of ability to cope. Human behavior has been assigned endless levels of meaning. Everyone is an amateur therapist: teachers, nurses, social workers, bartenders, pastors, and priests. Psychology has been reduced to a lifestyle.

Our society is engaged in a never-ending search for "normality" or "mental health." Psychiatrists and psychologists believe only they know what that is. Any deviation or natural problems of living stimulate analysis and speculations into the reasons why life is not idyllic. Mental health means tranquillity, peace of mind, happiness, and self-control. Look around you: Almost everyone has "problems." What is healthy and what is sick and who is to decide?

The psychological hierarchy endlessly reclassifies sick behavior and includes more and more individuals within the area of mental illness. Mental health authorities stand before audiences and proclaim: "Every family in America is touched by mental illness" or "One in four Americans has a mental problem." "Maladjustment" is the label they use to cover any of life's trials and tribulations. The psychological community promotes the concept that all malevolent behavior, all personal failure, most criminal acts, and most behavior problems would not have taken place if the individual had been well adjusted.

I recall one medical journal article two decades ago by a young psychiatrist who gave glowing promises for the future: "With our new psychological techniques, think of what we can do to aid the criminal justice system. . . ." And you know where the crime statistics have gone. "Think of what we can do for problem children. . . ." And you know the schools don't have problems with children anymore. "Think of what we can do to save marriages. . . ." You know the statistics on divorce.

Each graduating psychologist feels qualified to start his or her own school of therapy. Hundreds of books now in print by different authors describe the new healing methods each therapist promotes. The original purpose of psychology was to increase our sense of personal responsibility, but today it has done more to provide excuses for irresponsibility. We now have a good excuse for every naughty thing we do. Instead of giving our nation stability, psychology encourages us to question every decision our country makes. We trouble ourselves over every action we take. The tendency to see mental illness everywhere is a mistake for which we all pay the price. We speak of our most dangerous criminals as being "sick." Even though there is no proof this is true, guilt or innocence is determined less by *what* a person does, no matter how hideous the crime, than by *why* he did it. How he *felt* about what he did seems to determine his sentence.

Analyzing the analyzers

Two simple questions should always be asked about a psychologist's diagnosis: (1) Is it provable? and (2) Is it the *only* explanation?

The human mind forever falls into a universal trap: It cannot accept an event for which it has no ready explanation. To rid ourselves of our uneasiness in relation to the unknown we listen to any cleverly contrived answer to an unexplained phenomenon. Or we contrive our own explanation—anything to satisfy our need for a pat answer. We choose to believe what we *want* to believe.

I witnessed an experiment at a psychiatric hospital during which a subject was brought into a roomful of doctors for the purpose of demonstrating posthypnotic suggestion. Put into a trance, the patient was given a posthypnotic suggestion; upon awakening, he would not be able to open the door and leave the room nor would he remember the suggestion.

The patient was awakened and asked to go into the next room while the doctors consulted about his case. He approached the door but could not turn the knob. After several frustrating attempts, he gave up. One of the doctors insisted: "Would you please leave the room?"

Wrestling with his confusion, the patient replied: "I can't seem to turn the knob. It's probably because I hurt my hand yesterday."

Having no idea why he could not turn the knob, he *invented* a reason. His mind would not accept the lack of explanation for his behavior.

This is the trap into which many psychologists fall. They invent psychological explanations though there is no way to prove them. A *physiological* explanation, on the other hand, is not only provable but reproducible.

So many middle-class white therapists who work with ethnic lower-class groups try to understand their patients on the basis of a background of textbooks and classroom lectures, to no avail. They cannot truly know what the others are experiencing and feeling. The reason Alcoholics Anonymous has achieved greater success with problem drinkers than psychiatrists or religious zealots have is that each member has lived as the other member has lived. Each *knows* what the other is talking about. In the words of the Native American: "Do not judge me until you have walked a mile in my moccasins." Pointing out the trail is simply not the same as having traveled the trail.

The psychologist's view of cravings

Most psychologists lump craving problems under impulsive behavior and are content to suggest how to handle it. Sometimes they apply admonitions such as "You're going to have to try harder" or "Use your willpower." If they are more charitable they may say, "We need to find the real reasons behind these desires; once you know why you crave that particular food you will be able to stop craving it" or "Try substitute foods . . . take up a hobby . . . learn self-hypnosis" and so on. These are the traditional remedies that readers of this book have found totally unsatisfactory. Unfortunately these methods do not remove the cravings.

The psychologist feels that emotions control cravings. The logical treatment, then, is to eliminate the cravings by eliminating the mood that causes them. There are at least four reasons why this classic view is totally unfounded:

1. Many patients with cravings are perfectly normal people who often are under normal stresses, such as job pressures, interpersonal problems, or financial problems. There is no evidence whatsoever that their cravings signify some underlying mental disorder.

2. Anxiety, apprehension, frustration, and stress are normal reactions over which no one can expect to gain total control. These are defensive responses to the environment elicited by the body to relieve pressure. No amount of psychological therapy can stop this natural process.

3. Some people are genetically programmed to overrespond. They can't help overreacting to their environment, and they always will. If their particular programming includes craving food, then they will crave food.

4. The cravings of neurotics and psychotics are just as

likely to originate from physical motives as the cravings of normal people are. No amount of drug therapy can relieve them of their cravings. Even when they are cured of their mental disease, they will continue to crave.

The physical approach

The physical approach to cravings is in many ways the reverse of the classic approach. First, cravings are blocked by using the methods delineated in this book. Next, the anxiety symptoms associated with allergic withdrawal (cravings) cease to occur; as a result, the patient becomes less moody. Suppose you are hypoglycemic and are craving sugar. Consuming sugar will alleviate your moodiness and depression only temporarily. Controlling cravings by supplementation and *thereby* controlling anxiety is a better alternative than trying to control the cravings by controlling the anxiety that supposedly causes them.

Behavior modification therapy has no discernible effect on cravings. Neither does psychoanalysis, hypnosis, group therapy, aversion therapy, drug therapy, or any other kind of psychological intervention. Some psychologists might argue that allergy and deficiency as causes of cravings have not been fully accepted by the medical community. On the other hand, there has been no proof that cravings are psychological.

You may take your choice, but remember that *the proof is in the treatment*. Offering relatively immediate relief from the physical approach holds out a lot more hope for patients than telling them that someday, when treatment is successful, the hoped-for relief will come.

One note of hope—many mental health professionals are changing their tune. They are accepting nutritional methods and integrating them into their practices. They are leading the scientific community to better methods. You may be lucky enough to find one in your area. A guide for finding such practitioners can be found at the back of this book.

Strengths in the psychological approach

In behavior modification it is assumed that most socially relevant behavior is learned and reinforced through interactions with people and places. According to this view, the environment seems more important than the individual in determining behavior. Therefore, changing the environment would be the best way to change behavior.

If you want to improve your eating habits, here are some rules that will lead to much-needed changes. If these methods seem like a lot of trouble, ask yourself how much trouble you are willing to go to. Succeeding requires effort on your part. No pain, no gain.

1. Let each person in the family be responsible for getting his or her own food between meals. You can thereby reduce the number of times you come into contact with food. Getting food for others often means one for them and two for you.
2. Count the number of times you come into contact with food each day. Make up a list of the circumstances, then decide how many of these food confrontations you can avoid and find ways to do so.
3. Reduce the amount of importance you give to food. Don't talk about food to others. When you catch yourself thinking of food, immediately switch to other thoughts, no matter how many times you must do so. You might keep a count of the number of food thoughts you have each day for one week; in the second week, try to cut that number by half. This way, at least, you can prevent thoughts from triggering cravings.
4. Before you cook dinner, try two methods of staving off the hungries:

   a. Buy an empty eyedrop bottle or find yourself a nose-spray bottle. Put 1 teaspoon of vitamin C powder in four ounces of water and let it soak for half an hour. Pour the diluted vitamin C into the container and either drop several drops into each nostril or spray it into both sides of the nose several times. This can block the odors that switch on cravings.

  b. Eat one or two ounces of tuna with salt on it half
 an hour *before* you start to prepare dinner.
5. Repeat the "tuna technique" before you go food shopping. There is a definite reduction in "wrong" food
 purchases if you are not hungry in advance.
6. Don't cook or eat excessive amounts of food.
7. Make small portions seem larger.
8. Don't skip meals and wait until you're starved; feeling
 deprived may provoke more irresistible hunger than
 you can handle.
9. Plan regular meals and *eat every one of them*.
10. Keep a list of nonfood activities to replace snacking.
11. Have nutritious foods available.
12. Make good food as attractive as possible.
13. Eat slowly.
14. Keep the negative aspects of overeating in mind.
15. Exercise regularly.

As you can see, this is a formidable list of rules, but the
approach can help if you're up to it. If you'd like to learn
more, you can usually find a behavior modification class at
a local college or university in your area. There are also many
private psychologists who offer group sessions on behavior
modification. The granddaddy of books on the subject is *Slim
Chance in a Fat World—The Behavioral Control of Obesity*
by Richard B. Stewart (Research Press, 1972). It's a classic
and still in print.

Here is another technique I have found rather successful:
Make a list of the times and situations when you are likely
to eat too much or trigger your cravings. Find a comfortable
place at home to sit. It must be at a time when you won't be
disturbed. Close your eyes and rehearse what you think will
happen, imagining the entire period when your cravings could
be triggered.

For example, if the difficult time is Saturday afternoon
when your family is home, then quickly run through that
four-hour period and make a mental note of times and places
where your cravings start. Then re-think the same afternoon,
substituting new, better responses. This technique stimulates
you to come up with some solution for each problem time.

Then, when the real problem arises, you already know how to handle it. Thinking through a situation takes only five to ten minutes, and there are always good results.

The most important weapon against craving is *attitude*. If your attitude is poor, you had better attend to that as your first order of business. Bad attitudes stand in the way of competency. Avoid negative thinking and get past the complaining stage to the clean-up-the-problem stage. Once you have identified the problem, it's time to do something about it.

But remember, only *you* can make any of these techniques work. No one else will do it for you. And don't just talk about doing it. Talk is cheap. Action is victory.

CHAPTER FOURTEEN

Triggers to Hunger

A *hunger trigger* is a stimulus that induces a high enough level of excitement in the body to arouse the need or desire to eat. How and why we decide to eat is a subject of great interest to everyone today, especially the food industry. A great many signals trigger our feeding behavior, which is not surprising considering that all life forms must eat to survive. All organisms require energy. They must obtain food, eat, digest, and then repeat the process all over again to maintain energy and repair their bodies. Hunger is triggered both from inside and outside the body, and we and other animals enjoy not only what we need but what we don't need.

Hypoglycemia

One of the most publicized and overrated causes of cravings is hypoglycemia, or low blood sugar. This condition has become a popular topic among the general public and a source of controversy in the medical community. Some doctors have overemphasized its importance, while others deny that any such disease exists.

Body tissues need a continuous supply of food in order to function, and the body will burn sugar before it burns fat.

Therefore, blood sugar (glucose) is the predominant source of energy for all cells, but particularly for brain cells. The body's reserve of this immediately usable blood sugar is not sufficient to sustain the body for more than a few hours. When this supply is gone, it must be renewed by newly ingested foods or by a breakdown of body fat and/or protein from the basic tissues.

Hunger can be triggered when the blood sugar drops below a certain level. High levels of insulin in the circulation lower the sugar level and, most important, stimulate hunger. During my psychiatric residency, I witnessed patients who went on hunger strikes and refused to eat. Their will to fast was broken by injections of insulin, which lowered their blood sugar level and induced stomach contractions. They immediately became hungry and were compelled to eat. On the other hand, sugar injected directly into the bloodstream will *decrease* hunger contractions and yet will enhance the desire to eat. Diabetics, who are unable to metabolize sugar properly, may have high blood sugar levels and still be famished because their tissues are being deprived of nourishment.

Appetite suppressors such as amphetamine and atropine can block the hunger-triggering effects of insulin, even when the blood sugar level is very low. Large amounts of sugar in the blood can stimulate a considerable release of insulin from the pancreas. The homeostatic mechanisms must then distribute other hormones to suppress or compensate for the excessive amounts of insulin. If this occurs repeatedly, the cells' response to insulin is blunted and they become insulin resistant. In susceptible people, hypoglycemia can lead to one form of diabetes—adult-onset, or type II.

Varying stress factors can trigger hypoglycemia by releasing a neurotransmitter called beta-endorphin. Like caffeine, this hormone stimulates the pancreas to release insulin. Allergic reactions can trigger the symptoms of hypoglycemia or may even create the disease itself. Hunger and cravings, especially for carbohydrates, are known to occur when hypoglycemia is present.

The theory that the level of sugar in the blood directly causes cravings has been shown to be invalid. Hunger does not relate to the level of sugar in the blood but to the *intake* of sugar from the blood by the tissue cells. If it is slow, there is hunger; if fast, there is satiety. If blood of recently fed animals is transferred to hungry animals, it tends to decrease their hunger by 50 percent, indicating that a chemical substance circulating in the blood after eating signals the brain's "appestat" to switch to "off."

In one experiment, rats were artificially joined so that their blood supply mingled like that of Siamese twins. The "twin" that ate second always ate 20 to 30 percent less food than the twin that ate first, no matter how the researchers alternated the feeding pattern. In another experiment the researchers destroyed the hypothalamus of one of each pair of joined rats. This part of the brain controls feeding behavior. The "twin" with no feeding "regulator" ate constantly and became obese. Its "twin" became thinner and thinner. Apparently, a "satisfaction signal" was present in the blood of the overeating, obese rat, even though its brain could not respond to the signal. This chemical was signaling the *normal* rat's brain to stop feeding behavior. In other words, the more the fat rat ate, the less its "twin" ate.

Whether or not you are hypoglycemic is a matter of your blood sugar level. In individual cases, hypoglycemia may or may not cause cravings. Other factors are involved besides blood sugar, which may affect different people differently. Whether blood sugar or some other factor signals hunger or satiety to the brain, bear in mind that *many* factors combine to affect hunger.

Sugar as a drug

Sugar destroys your body's delicate chemical balance. When you consume simple sugars like table sugar, candy, or colas, they pass directly to the intestines to be converted to glucose. Because they are absorbed so rapidly into the bloodstream, these sugars upset a precise balance and drastically increase the glucose level. To counteract this imbalance, insulin rushes in to lower the glucose level while adrenal hormones work double-time to raise it. These mechanisms are in direct conflict with each other. As a result, the pancreas, which produces insulin, and the adrenal glands are overworked, causing havoc to the endocrine system.

The effect is immediate: At first you feel "up," until the bottom drops out from under your blood sugar level. Then you experience fatigue and listlessness. You can become nervous and irritable, your brain vulnerable to suspicion and distrust. Your efficiency lags, and you can't handle stress because your endocrine circuits are too out of balance to cope with it.

Far from being nutritional, simple sugar is a poison that can cause a drug-like effect when overconsumed. Too much of it can send shock waves to your system. Lab experiments with rats have shown that excessive doses of sugar can be toxic enough to cause death.

Sugar is an antinutrient. It provides nothing but empty calories. Worse, it drains vitamins and minerals from your body because digestion, detoxification, and elimination of sugar require large amounts of nutrients.

In small amounts, natural sugars like those in fruit and potatoes are good for energy and do not disturb body balances. Heavy doses of sugar in concentrated form act as a toxin to the body. The stress from its use is not immediately dangerous but, over the years, it causes considerable damage. In the end it can become life threatening.

One way to stabilize blood sugar levels is the use of the trace element chromium. Chromium makes body cells more receptive to insulin, stabilizing the blood glucose level and thereby reducing cravings. To make use of this effect, you can purchase brewer's yeast tablets from the health food store and take them daily. Brewer's yeast is high in chromium. Remember that if you are a diabetic or have some other chronic disease, you should not try this without your doctor's knowledge and consent.

If you are hypoglycemic, you should not eat refined sugar but should stick to unrefined starches such as whole grains, beans, and brown rice. Most protocols for hypoglycemia also recommend six small meals a day. Six meals a day can become quite a burden, so I recommend a substitute snack: Use a small serving of protein with salt on it during any "drop off" time.

Female hormones as hunger triggers

Many women report cravings, binge eating, or higher levels of hunger just before their menstrual period. Studies have clearly demonstrated that female hormones affect hunger. Both estrogen and progesterone levels in the average woman fluctuate during the monthly cycle. An imbalance in these levels can increase or decrease hunger. Unfortunately, women often receive bad advice from doctors who dismiss their physiological cravings as psychological—despite scientific studies to the contrary. Unlike other types of cravings, those related to female hormone imbalance cannot be self-corrected. *Consult your family physician or call one of the organizations listed herein.*

Other hunger-triggering hormones

Excesses or deficiencies of all human hormones can alter feeding behavior. High doses of male hormones such as testosterone decrease appetite; low doses stimulate appetite. Increased thyroid activity can increase hunger.

Patients report an increase in cravings under stress, especially long or difficult stress (a time when food cravers can develop hormone deficiency). Those who have had multiple stresses can become relatively deficient in cortisone, especially if the adrenal glands are not healthy to start with.

Patients who use a lot of drugs often overwork the adrenal glands, leading to adrenal insufficiency. Cortisone by prescription increases hunger and water retention and hence body weight. Almost all patients given prolonged doses of cortisone gain weight; much of the fat is distributed to the torso. Even worse, cortisone causes the craving by enhancing taste; it changes the chemical composition of saliva.

What can one do about this group of stimulators to cravings? Use the pantothenic acid supplements as described in the chapters on salt cravings. This will help with hunger that relates to the adrenal glands. Male hormone imbalances must be treated by your personal physician.

Fat hormones. Recent research has closely tied food intake to prostaglandins. These hormones, which are produced in body fat, convey information to the brain about fat tissue content.

In general, excesses or deficiencies of almost every known human hormone can affect your hunger or cravings for certain foods.

Chewing

The need for oral *stimulation* and oral *satisfaction* is universal. The process of chewing produces a feeling of fullness, thereby removing the sensation of hunger. How many times have you felt like putting something into your mouth even though you're not physically hungry? Food placed directly in the stomach through a tube will not relieve hunger without the oral satisfaction of chewing.

The opposite is also true—food chewed and spat out will not completely relieve hunger. Some food must enter the stomach. A full stomach reduces the response to the smell and taste of food.

Taste

Taste can cause overeating. The better a food tastes, of course, the more you will eat. Most people can still have dessert on a full stomach. The desire for sugary food overrides the body's satisfaction signals. Taste can also change mealtimes. Rats are nocturnal eaters, but if a tasty food is available, they will give up their nocturnal instincts and become daytime eaters.

Intestinal signals

Feelings of hunger do not necessarily rely on stomach contractions. Even people whose stomachs are removed feel hunger. In addition, when the nerves to the stomach are cut, hunger sensations still occur, even though sensations from the stomach are not transmitted to the brain.

The small intestine usually gets a small sample of food from the stomach a few minutes after the meal. The rest of the food stays in the stomach to be digested. If the food from one meal is still being digested and a second meal is eaten, the stomach will send a small amount of the second meal to the small intestine for sampling even though the food from the first meal is still being digested. The stomach has its own "intelligence." It sends on samples from each new meal, especially those containing mostly sugar and carbohydrates. Since the most powerful signals of satisfaction come from the small intestine, the mind is signaled to stop eating. Under healthy conditions, this intestinal sampling helps the body determine food intake.

Many times we eat compulsively without thinking. We're semiconscious of what we're doing, but we ignore the stop-eating signals. Since these signals take ten to fifteen minutes to reach our brains, we may gulp down an entire meal before the signals tell us we are full.

When sugar is placed directly into the small intestine through a tube, there is at least a five-minute delay in fullness signaling. This has led researchers to believe that satisfaction signals are not due to blood sugar increases, but possibly due to a satiety hormone in the small intestine called cholecystokinin. This hormone is present for only ten to fifteen minutes before it disappears from the blood.

Most overweight people feel that, once they have lost weight and their stomach has "shrunk," they will be less likely to overeat. Granted, the stretch receptors in the stomach walls are now more sensitive than when it had been ingesting larger meals, but when the person begins to overeat again, these stretch receptors become less sensitive to greater amounts of food.

A candy sold in drug stores is designed to "spoil" meals. If you take it 45 minutes before eating, it will supposedly raise the blood sugar level and provide the necessary stop-eating signals. To a limited degree this technique works. The trouble is that eating enough candy to reduce hunger can become a self-defeating effort. I have, however, seen many people use this technique very successfully to reduce hunger and cravings.

Stomach condition.   The general health of your stomach can substantially increase your level of hunger. For example, excess acid irritates the stomach and promotes hunger; the presence of a hiatus hernia brings on a sense of emptiness and insatiability. The vagus nerve can overstimulate the stomach and cause perpetual hunger.

Aloe vera juice is an excellent way to calm the stomach. Keep a bottle in the refrigerator at home and use one or two ounces if you feel you need to eat to neutralize stomach acid pains.

Erroneous signals from the stomach

Hunger among the overweight varies from person to person. Intense hunger may cause one person to overeat; for another, the problem may be a disorganization of the signaling system. People may feel like eating without being hungry. They have no idea when they are hungry, because there is no light on the dashboard; the feeling of hunger has not reached a level of awareness.

Though many overweight people do not complain of actual hunger, they behave as if they were *always* hungry. They usually overeat at every meal, particularly dinner, devouring their food like famine victims, their taste buds in high gear.

Intestinal bypass surgery may temporarily reverse this self-destructive process. But my experience with dozens of bypass patients is that after five years or so, the cravings return with a vengeance.

Compare the behavior of an overweight man with that of a genuinely starving man. Both have heightened taste responsiveness; both tend to crave carbohydrates. Neither is more responsive to normal feeding cues than the other. Both are less active and, generally, have low sexual inclinations. The obese male experiences the same signals as that of a starved man, but not the same as the normal male.

These erroneous signals are caused by metabolic imbalances that cannot be changed by today's treatment methods. One way to work around this would be to deal directly with your eating behavior per se. Start treating yourself as though you *are* hungry. If you want to eat but don't feel hungry, act as though you are in fact very hungry. Then use any of the previously mentioned techniques for craving control.

Thirst and hunger

Another important cause of hunger is the retention of *body water*. Water is required for proper metabolism, so the regulation of food and water intake are closely related. I have observed innumerable patients whose thirst increases along with their hunger.

If you drink eight or ten glasses of water a day, you will experience less hunger, not because your stomach is filled with water but rather because of the effect of overhydration on the hunger-thirst center. Bottled water is preferable to tap water, which is too contaminated with chemicals. If done diligently, drinking water becomes a good habit. Eight glasses of water a day is considered to be an essential part of any good health program. Other beverages don't count.

Drugs that trigger hunger

Tranquilizers, cortisone, and a number of antihistamines are among the commonly used drugs that have been known to increase hunger. The use of marijuana increases cravings, and alcohol consumption alters hunger patterns. Lithium stimulates hunger by increasing insulin levels.

The worst offenders are insulin and oral antidiabetic drugs, heavy-duty tranquilizers, and strong antidepressants. If you must use prescription drugs, you have little choice. But ask your doctor about changing to lesser doses or to less appetite-stimulating drugs.

Smoking

Nicotinic acid affects the level of insulin. Those who have stopped smoking usually experience an increase in insulin levels that can produce a weight gain of as much as twenty pounds for the average person. Insulin is also a powerful water retainer; hence the connection between withdrawal of tobacco use and increased hunger. Weight gain when ceasing to smoke involves more than just psychological factors.

Fatigue and insomnia

Both fatigue and insomnia stimulate hunger. Restless sleepers eat more to keep up their energy level to get through the day. Tired people who are overweight tend to eat more when their energy level is down. Fatigue means an unbalanced body which, as we have seen, can be a very powerful trigger to cravings. I have helped certain patients lose weight by prescribing not a diet pill but a sleeping pill. In such cases, hunger and cravings are wholly related to insomnia.

To treat insomnia yourself, you have a wide choice of sleep-inducing herbs from the health food store. Try three tablets of the herb valerian or Sleepytime tea just before bedtime.

If energy is the problem, try four liver tablets four times a day, but not too close to bedtime. Add 100 mg vitamin B_6 three times a day, again not near bedtime. Nutro-Homo powder from Bioresearch in Redondo Beach, California, is also an excellent energy boost that will decrease hunger rather than cause it. Use one tablespoonful twice a day. Fatigue is a multiheaded monster with far too many causes to deal with here.

Vitamins and foods can be triggers

Another trigger to hunger is vitamin supplements, which may unbalance your body. Frequently I hear patients say, "I had to stop taking 'X' vitamin because it increased my hunger.'' Vitamins that properly complement your body should actually *decrease* hunger. Natural foods are balanced in essential nutrients, which means that it is not hard to obtain a healthy diet. Most individuals fortunately require novelty. This encourages them to eat more than one food during a meal and to seek variety in tastes. In this general way health can be maintained.

On the negative side, if the food has a highly rewarding quality to it—i.e., pleasurable taste, odor, and texture—and, in addition, gives hunger and tension relief (withdrawal symptoms), we have a setup for cravings.

Individual preferences for food are both characteristic of the individual and reflective of the metabolic state at the time. Variations in taste sensitivity also affect preferences. In both animals and people there are wide individual variations in the ''set'' of the hedonistic mechanisms.

In 1957, G. W. Wharton noted that many animals whose diet consists of large amounts of vegetation may seek to increase their mineral intake by eating dirt. Eating earth as a way to mineral balance is a natural phenomenon, not a sign of mental disturbance.

Jane Goodall (1963) says that chimpanzees in Africa eat vegetables but also insects and meat. She saw them eat blossoms, seeds, and bark ants, termites, caterpillars, bee larvae, birds' eggs, and small birds. They killed bush bucks, pigs, young baboons, and monkeys. Interestingly, they ate mouthfuls of leaves along with the meat to provide proper mineral balance.

Nutro-Homo by Bioresearch is an excellent example of a completely balanced vitamin that will decrease hunger rather than cause it. If your vitamins are making you hungry, use another formulation.

Chemical allergies

Chemicals may also trigger hunger. While testing patients for chemical allergies, I discovered that a number of patients became hungry or craved particular foods after exposure to gasoline, chlorine, or petrochemicals. One patient, a swimming instructor, craved sugars after exposure to chlorine. She made the connection between the constant munchies she gets when poolside and an allergy to chlorine. Another allergic patient reported hunger while doing the laundry: chlorine again. A third patient was found to be allergic to auto exhaust fumes; hunger was her typical reaction. Driving in her car, she would develop irresistible urges to eat.

Be aware of the possible relationship your cravings may have to chemicals. They are extremely difficult to treat. It's best to seek professional help.

Weather and hunger

An often overlooked cause of hunger is body temperature in relation to environment. We eat more in cold weather than in warm weather because extra food is required to maintain body heat. In a study of combat infantrymen in the field, soldiers consumed an average of 5,000 calories per day when the temperature was minus 40 degrees Fahrenheit. Their consumption dropped to 3,000 calories per day when the temperature rose to plus 100 degrees Fahrenheit.

When there is a sudden heat wave, our food intake often drops. After we adjust to the change in weather, it shoots back up again. It is believed that high environmental temperatures lower our "setpoint," i.e., the regulatory system that maintains our body weight.

Research evidence has shown that twenty minutes a day of exposure to lowered temperatures is enough to produce an increase in food intake. So a cold environment does in fact increase the motivation to eat. And the older you are, the more your body responds to this condition.

Your body's ability to survive cold temperatures also increases when the food you eat is richer in fats and carbohydrates. When the weather becomes colder you may respond by eating more foods that contain sugar, oil, and butter.

Many people with arthritis notice they can tell when the weather is going to change by the numbers of aches and pains that they register. One good explanation for this is mold infection. For example, I treated a young child who had had diarrhea for several years. It usually happened just before a rainstorm. At that time there are many more mold spores in the air than usual. Normally, the typical spore count in the air ranges from 200 to 300 per unit of volume. Just before it rains, however, there is a moisture change. Then the mold spores in the same volume of air can be thirty to forty *thousand*. This can happen in a matter of only 60 minutes.

Increased appetite during cold, damp weather is often blamed on the need for extra calories to fight off cold. This is no doubt an arguable cause. However, hunger can also stem from an accentuation of a mold allergy.

Psychological triggers

Under natural conditions, self-selection of foods has always been a healthy instinct. But in response to the artificial stimulations present in modern society, self-selection tends to go awry. Not only are we bombarded by fast-food advertisements, we are stigmatized from birth by social and ethnic behavior patterns that adversely influence our hunger cycles. By today's standards, these hunger patterns are considered the norm, so their extension into the pathological range is quite understandable. Suffice it to say that our mental state can trigger irrepressible urges to eat, driving us to levels of hunger and cravings that willpower alone can't touch.

A common statement made by my overweight patients is that they have total control over the rest of their lives, but this is one area where they seem to be absolutely helpless. They demonstrate consistently good disciplinary patterns in almost every aspect of daily life—except for hunger and cravings. Another statement I hear constantly: "Every time I get upset I can't stop eating," or "When I get upset, boy! do I start to crave things." Without question, psychological events do trigger cravings.

In this chapter I have tried to present an overview of the many triggers to hunger. More exist than have been included here, but the sampling is enough to make the point.

If we tried to block all the possible triggers to hunger and cravings, we would not have time in a lifetime for anything else. Our best approach is to neutralize the cravings when they start, regardless of the trigger. And above all, we must take preventive action to control allergy and yeast problems where they exist. These are by far the factors most responsible for the majority of cravings.

CHAPTER FIFTEEN

Hunger as a Business

No one could profess to know more about craving and hunger than the kingpins on Madison Avenue. They mastered the art of manipulating cravings long before doctors ever speculated about it. In fact, the control of cravings rests in their hands and they exercise it skillfully to multiply their handsome profits.

The Madison Avenue experts say . . .

According to one advertising source, the average American receives *two thousand* advertising messages per day. A goodly number of those relate to food. No one can deny that the visual effect of a billboard or TV commercial depicting food acts to trigger our hunger.

If insulin is injected into your body, its effect will lower your blood sugar and precipitate an increase in hunger. Similarly, if pictures of appetizing foods are flashed before you, your insulin level automatically rises and your blood sugar goes down. You get the munchies.

Madison Avenue's audiovisual stimulation of our cravings is all-pervasive. We cannot turn on a television, open a magazine, or jog down the block without running into food advertisements. With voices cooing over donut delights and romantic images of two forks and one wedge of cheesecake seducing us, how can we ever expect to control ourselves?

Not only do the ads affect us, but the sights and smells of food from refreshment stands and places of entertainment bombard us everywhere. The food industry has planned it that way. Theaters make their revenue, not from ticket sales, but from the concession stand. Popcorn and candy offer bigger profits than the movie or play. Even opera houses and concert halls now have food bars; the managements have learned that revenue is better than snobbery. Social contacts, from parties to business lunches, inevitably involve food.

Many meals in the United States are eaten away from home. These meals are often prepackaged by highly competitive companies that spend millions in research to find new ways —often with new forms of sugar—to improve the taste appeal of their foods. With all these sugar traps, how can we keep from being ensnared in their alluring webs? It is difficult indeed to resist all these obstacles that physiologically and psychologically block our way to good health. But knowledge is our best weapon and, with heightened awareness of the food industry's seductive influence, we can find ways to fight back.

The food industry spends hundreds of millions of dollars a year to condition us into being obedient consumers like Pavlov's dogs. The more it spends, the more we eat. No one can match the food industry in manipulating society with the high art of behavior modification. They lead all other advertising business in consumer response to ads (Figure 1). The cola industry is doubling in size every two years, fast foods every three years. Every day of the year, McDonald's opens two more burger stands.

I think when astronauts land on Mars, the first thing they'll see is a pair of golden arches. I remember once looking out my hotel-room window in Kowloon across the bay to Hong Kong Island. The lights along the waterfront shimmered with exotic beauty. So did the huge golden arches of McDonald's. I have seen those arches in South America, Japan, Europe, Africa, everywhere. Yes, isn't it nice to get away?

The food industry is the major contributor to "setting off"

Figure 1

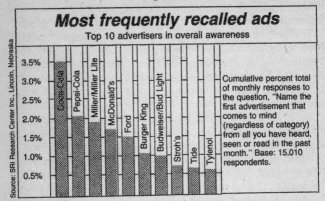

Reprinted with permission from the January 30, 1984, issue of *Advertising Age*. Copyright 1984 by Crain Communications, Inc.
Source: SRI Research Center, Inc., Lincoln, Nebraska.

our triggers of craving and hunger. Much of the industry's megabucks are spent on researching hunger-triggering "impulse items" such as candy placed at eye level near the cash register. Once our buttons have been pushed, our body chemistry alters, so that we may have to fight off cravings for a good part of an hour. If our buttons are pushed countless times a day by subtle design, inevitably our resistance will break down.

Some individuals are primed for these advertising triggers whose impulses can be set off like explosive charges. They already have physical craving problems to start with, due to food allergies, candidiasis, or deficiencies. The food industry harvests this crop of consumers on a daily basis.

Food technologists take "purchase resistance" very seriously. They assign panels of consumer specialists to achieve an "optimization of sensory attributes," and improve "the desire to obtain" through high-level sensory appeal. Food evaluations are determined by extensive consumer testing. Word-association tests are used to determine which words motivate people to buy—words like "creamy," "fudgy," "finger-lickin' good" or phrases like "Bet ya can't eat just one." Such messages are mathematically rated in terms of consumer impact, calculated to see which inspire the most colorful images in the mind's eye. An entire new science related to foods, in fact, is devoted to studying the consumer to help the food industry capitalize on its findings.

Consumatory behavior and instinct

An instinctual urge is a random searching behavior with a specific purpose: the release of energy. With this urge comes a hierarchy of needs. We direct all our attention and energy toward whatever perceived need might exist at that moment, following a kind of mechanical program given to us by nature.

A second aspect of instinct is appetite behavior, a desire and striving for satisfaction in attaining our instinctual goal. The intensely strong need to consummate our appetite is, in itself, an innate instinct. It often overbalances the physical need of homeostasis, each at cross purposes with the other. One purpose may be to satisfy an appetite, which comes into conflict with another goal, losing weight. Once a need for a substance is satisfied, a body with a properly balanced homeostasis and appetite control communicates this fulfillment to the pleasure centers. As a result, a dislike for that substance should develop.

One way this is manifested is by our need for novelty. Boredom at eating the same foods brings on a need for a taste change. ("Chinese food or Mexican food tonight?") And yet many people have favorite foods which they overuse or abuse. An unobstructed, excessive consumption of the same food because it's easily available may often lead to a reactive-allergic addiction.

By its general nature, consumatory behavior may subvert many conflicting psychological and physical needs. The satisfaction of our psychological needs may be sought after to the detriment of our physical needs. The difficulty in managing consumatory behavior is that once an appetite has been started and energized, there is a powerful need to finish the action, to get a sense of completion, to close the curtain.

Living "high off the hog" can enhance the high-volume consumer's social status, thereby providing more opportunities to buy, stockpile, and consume a particular food product. This unending supply assures well-to-do consumers that they need never be deprived of their instinctual need.

Of all highly developed life forms, we humans are the most influenced by pleasure. Pleasure motivation has changed our pattern of consumatory behavior from one of homeostatic balance of bodily needs to one of sensory comsumption, with detrimental results.

This peculiar phenomenon of satisfying sensory needs is not indigenous to humans alone. Many animals will throw caution to the winds to attain pleasure. Laboratory rats will suffer great pain to cross electrically charged grids in order to reach a cube of sugar. The danger to man is that he has a far greater ability to invent and discover unlimited paths to pleasure. This relentless pursuit of pleasure can seriously disturb the vital energy balance of the human body.

So, we must discover and invent new ways to restrain our excessive desires for sensory pleasure. Self-restraint can take various forms, such as the submission to moral and peer pressures.

The consumatory pleasure and fulfillment of satisfying an appetite often lead to a sense of emptiness. Food is not the only source of pleasure, though the food industry would like you to think so. Consumatory behavior has become such a major preoccupation in our society that we sometimes overlook other satisfying activities such as peaceful contemplation, unmotivated behavior, or spontaneous play, which all contribute to a better psychological and homeostatic balance.

Sensory temptations

The food industry has countless ways to manipulate the sensory aspects of its products. How food looks, smells, and tastes can be a primary force in motivating "buying behavior."

Color. The first appearance of a food is an important factor toward triggering hunger. Unappetizing appearance will affect its flavor and taste. Using food colors to excite consumer interest is a major concern to food technologists and optical engineers.

The purple color of fresh meat, for example, derives from an iron pigment. Once exposed to air, meat turns red. Whether the meat is light or dark depends on the concentration of pigment and the amount of reflected light. Animal species, age, and nutritional state before death affect color; so does the carcass's rate of cooling. The amount of stress during slaughter can modify the translucency or opaqueness of the meat. Above all, the attractiveness of the market's illuminated display can influence the meat's colors. Light can make all the difference between profit and loss.

Taste.   The tongue can distinguish four taste qualities: sweet, sour, salty, and bitter. It is the combination of the qualities that determine taste. Condiments and flavoring agents mixed together can change taste, even though there is no actual chemical reaction between the different ingredients. But the taste sensors do not recognize each component to the same degree.

Novelty in taste is an important aspect of marketing food products. Food technologists diligently manipulate the consistency of foods to breathe some excitement into them. A little scientific ingenuity can go a long way. In chocolate manufacturing, sugar crystals can be controlled by size and distribution, as can the ratio of milk to fat, the moisture content, and the amount of fibrous cocoa material.

The primary goal of all this sensory analysis and manipulation of product is enhancing public acceptance. The most effective means to this end is today's sensory temptation without peer, the food industry's long-time ace in the hole: sugar. No food substance is more addicting.

Sweets: The real enemy

Sweetness motivates people to select carbohydrates over other food. In nature, selecting sweet fruits over unripe, sour fruits is valuable both to personal survival and to species survival.

Ripe fruits have more nutrients. This preference for sweetness is built into all of us, although carbohydrate hunger seems to be greater in women—both in frequency of desire and degree of hunger.

To cater to our taste for sweets, today's cattle are often fed sugar prior to slaughter to improve their flavor. Molasses blended with corn syrup may be added to a restaurant's hamburger meat. Or perhaps you prefer a fish filet. Watch out for the breading: It's loaded with sugar. An order of fries? Raw potato slices are often dipped in sugar solutions before they are deep-fried. How about that chicken stand? Careful; most processed chicken is injected with honey or other sugars before frying.

You're just a big sugar cube

Every year the average American knowingly or unknowingly consumes sugar equivalent to the size of an entire human body. Because of the abundance of sugar in commercial products and the unintentional overuse of "hidden sugars" by the unwary, it is exceedingly difficult to avoid sugar consumption, which only triggers the desire for more sugar.

Sugars are easily recognizable in processed sweets and prepared desserts. But they are barely discernible in many other foods. Concealed sweeteners are present in a disheartening array of products, particularly the popular convenience foods so prevalent in our society. For example, catsup contains more sugar per ounce than ice cream. Many salad dressings have three times the sugar content of cola drinks, and some nondairy creamers have more sugar than a chocolate bar. From cigarettes to cottage cheese, at home, market, restaurant, or vending machine, you cannot escape sugar.

Manufacturers use many guises to deceive the consumer about the ingredients in a product. One of the most misleading labels on these products is "natural carbohydrates." You may be a committed label-watcher, but often in the supermarket you will look at an ingredient list that reads: "Wheat, vegetable oil, dextrose, corn syrup solids, and malt powder."

The last three ingredients are pure sugar. They are listed separately to avoid listing sugar as the main ingredient. Yet if you were buying a grain product, this would be the equivalent of asking a waitress for a little cereal to sprinkle on your bowl of sugar.

Sweetness is not the only reason for the use of sugar in commercial foods. Molasses has the ability to mask certain unpleasant flavors such as the bitter taste in bran. It can also mimic the flavors of chocolate, butterscotch, coffee, and maple and is sometimes added to enhance these natural flavors. Molasses also reduces the rate of food spoilage because of its antioxidant effect, especially when mixed with starch, flour, or other kinds of sugar. These blends are used in bakery products, sausages, and even some health foods. Because the product is a molasses blend, its label may read only "molasses," omitting such items as corn, wheat, or soy, which may afflict the unsuspecting buyer with hidden allergies.

In some states, only 51 percent of a product need be derived from one source for that source's name to be printed on the label. Therefore, an item labeled as honey may in fact be a blend of starch, flour, sugar, and syrup used to change its color and increase its weight and texture. Take a look sometime at that bottle of "old-fashioned" New England/Vermont buttered maple syrup with its nostalgic-styled, "natural" label on the market shelf. In reality, it may contain very little if *any* maple syrup and may consist primarily of cane sugar boosted with artificial flavorings and coloring.

Another misleading ingredient is corn sweeteners. More than half of all cornstarch milled in America is converted into corn sugar and corn syrup. These products are further refined into glucose, maltose, and lump sugar. Less expensive than cane sugar, corn sugar is a low-cost sweetener for products contained in syrups such as canned fruits. The addition of corn syrup to sucrose and other sugars inhibits crystallization, which helps hold together confections like hard candy, jam, jelly, preserves, and ice cream. Since corn sweeteners are readily soluble, corn syrup also adds body and texture to your soft drink and pliability to your chewing gum.

The confection industry is not the only exploiter of corn

sweeteners. Dextrose readily ferments yeast and is used for this purpose by brewers, distillers, and bakers. Bakers find that dextrose contributes an attractive brown crust color and enhances the flavor of their product. It also inhibits undesirable oxidation of certain foods and helps retain bright colors in strawberry and peach preserves, cured meats, and catsup.

All these corn sweeteners highlight color and impart sheen to food surfaces, increasing their sales appeal. They absorb and retain moisture to keep candies from sticking and lollipops from dripping. But all they are doing for us is adding more varieties of poison to our daily diet.

A classic case of creative advertising is that of sugar-free gum. The "sugarless" sugar it contains is *sorbitol*, an artificial sweetener that has the same number of calories as regular sugar, only with a slower absorption rate. Natural sorbitol is found in berries, cherries, plums, apples, and blackstrap molasses. It was originally extracted from these natural fruits, but no longer. Today's commercial sorbitol is manufactured from our old sugary friend, glucose.

Sorbitol is a frequent additive for baked goods, frosting, gelatin puddings, dairy products, processed fish, poultry and meat, snack foods, fats, oils, alcoholic beverages, sauces, and seasonings. Sometimes it is used to coat baking goods to keep them from flaking or crumbling, other times as a lubricant on grill-cooked meats.

Mannitol, another so-called sugarless sugar, is used in the same manner as sorbitol but is also found in breath fresheners, antacid tablets, cough medicines, and children's aspirins.

The problem with these sugar substitutes is that they can produce the same ill effects as the items they are replacing. Some chemical sweeteners may have no calories but can stimulate hunger or cause addictive allergies. Their overall value is definitely *not* in the best interests of our physical health and well-being.

In addition to sugar-contaminated foods, we are further plagued by the wide use of sugar in such innocent nonfoods as drugs, cosmetics, and perfumes. As a filler, sugar can comprise a large portion of many drug tablets, capsules, and pills. However unavoidable they may be, here are some to watch out for:

adhesives	tapes	lubricants
envelopes	aspirin	ointments
stamps	bath powders	paper cups
dentifrices	body oils	suppositories
hair sprays	body powder	talcums
lozenges	breath sprays	toothpaste
stickers	cold remedies	wax

The tobacco industry has been increasing its use of refined sugar, which is added to air-cured tobacco during the blending process. This apparently improves the flavor and burning quality of the leaves. Extensive research has suggested that the increase in cancer from cigarettes may be attributed, in part, to the sugar content. The presence of sugar in cigarettes could also act as a trigger for hunger, although the nicotinic acid tends to nullify that effect. Either way, it is not worth the risk to smoke under any circumstances.

Chocolate: Montezuma's revenge

"The best things in life aren't free—they cost five dollars a pound." Succulent creams and silky-smooth, chocolate-covered delights make the saliva flow.

Chocolate is more a fix than a feast, as history will attest. The Aztec emperor Montezuma II was a committed chocophile who always served a chaliceful of his "chocolatl" love potion to break down the inhibitions of nubile Indian maidens recruited into his harem. It has been recorded that he tossed back fifty golden goblets a day—a true allergic addiction if ever there was one.

Theobroma cacao (Greek for "food for the gods") originated in the Amazon rain forests and the tropical wilds of Mexico. There bloomed the tropical evergreen, the cacao tree. According to legend the Aztec serpent god of the air, Quetzalcoatl, bestowed upon his people the gift of this tree which once only the immortals enjoyed: the sweet cacao fruit. At first he enjoined them to suck only the fruit itself, discarding the pod shell and the seeds. Then, in his great wisdom, he taught them to throw the seeds into a fire to give forth a rich and pleasurable aroma. When the seeds cooled, the Aztecs tasted them anew and discovered that they bore a delightfully rich new food which, when mixed with water, made an excellent drink.

For bringing so cherished a gift out of paradise for the pleasure of mere mortals, Quetzalcoatl was flayed alive by his fellow gods. But it was too late. Mankind had discovered the joy of chocolate.

In time, chocolate evolved into a form of currency. During tribal wars, huge quantities of cacao beans were surrendered by vanquished tribes as a tribute to their conquerors. Ten seeds could be bartered for a rabbit. A hundred could buy a slave. The services of an Indian woman could be procured for eight cacao beans a night, much the way soldiers in war-torn Europe traded chocolate bars for a night's pleasures.

America was not the only discovery made by Christopher Columbus. In 1502, on the coast of Nicaragua, he experienced his first taste of chocolate. But the bitter brew did not agree with him and he sailed on without it.

Seventeen years later Hernando Cortes made the same discovery, but his reaction was far different. Visiting Montezuma's palace, the Spanish conquistador was treated to this luxurious, dark-brown concoction, which the emperor savored like ambrosia.

Cortes found the emperor's "chocolatl" rank in taste but remarkable in effect; it gave him the strength to march all day long. He was so overwhelmed by it that the cacao bean was prominent among the gold and rich spoils he took back to Spain after his cruel, bloody conquest of the Aztecs. Considering the impact of the "brown curse" on chocolate addicts around the world today, chocolate, not *turista*, may be Montezuma's *true* revenge.

For more than a century, Spain kept the cultivation and preparation of chocolate a guarded national secret. But when Spanish and French royalty married in 1615, the beverage crossed the Pyrenees to the courts of France, where its stimulating effect eventually led to its staggering popularity among the nobility. Because of its reputation as an aphrodisiac, the Church condemned chocolate as the drink of the Devil. But once it was mixed with a new commodity called sugar, it proved unstoppable.

Before long, chocolate won over the Old and New Worlds like a Brown Plague of ooh's and ahh's and upset tummies. Sugared and spiced with nutmegs, cloves, lemon peel, and everything nice, it became the rage of Europe. Like our coffee shops today, chocolate houses became the fashion and were regularly frequented by the social aristocracy. The chocolate habit was deemed elegant and chic. Learned physicians extolled the medical virtues of this sweet elixir.

With the advent of chocolate shops came the expansion of chocolate plantations, which brought as much wealth as tobacco and slaves. The planting and cultivating of the cacao plant combined with the Industrial Revolution to bring on the first chocolate-processing factories.

Every chocolate factory praised its own secret formula. The invention of the solid chocolate bar changed the face of the confectionery world, but it was Hershey who brought it within reach of the common folk when he perfected an easy way to make milk chocolate and advertised his mass-produced Hershey bars on early American automobiles. And when a Swiss confectioner invented the process of conching, the texture of chocolate changed to make it what it is today: that irresistible melt-in-your-mouth smoothness.

The chocolate craze goes on, fortified by endless claims about its health benefits. Ever since Napolean supplied his ranks with chocolate for quick energy, front-line soldiers everywhere carry it with them as part of their battle rations. Mountain climbers keep it in their gear for that extra boost, as did Sir Edmund Hillary when he scaled Mount Everest. Chocolate has gone aboard space flights to maintain astronauts' energy levels at their peak. The aphrodisiac claims continue unchecked. Recently, a chemical found in chocolate called phenylethylalamine has been proclaimed the trigger that acts on the brain when people fall in love.

Chocolate has taken the modern world by storm. It is here to stay, with staggering profits to be made. Its glamour and appeal knows no bounds as new fads crop up: chocolate-molded T-shirts and ties, chocolate Monopoly games, chocolate-scented paper, chocolate tobacco, chocolate omelets, and chocolate chili.

Chocolate has become an institution. In 1980, two employees of the Swiss chocolate industry were arrested trying to sell to China and Russia some of their nation's most closely guarded secrets: forty recipes for making chocolate.

For millions of us, the "high" from that daily chocolate fix makes life bearable. There is no world shortage, so we don't have to share it if we don't want to. There is always tomorrow and more French chocolate mint truffles, Godiva chocolate strawberry creams, sour-cherry chocolate torte, Tobler Extra-Bittersweet, Hershey's Kisses, Dutch chocolate cheesecake ice cream, chocolate fondue, chocolate mousse, chocolate eclairs, chocolate napoleons, chocolate fudge sundaes, chocolate pinwheels, chocolate meringues, chocolate custard, chocolate creams, chocolate colas. . . .

The sugar curse

For five centuries the Sweet Tooth Fairy has been winning the sugar battle. Today, over a third of our daily carbohydrate consumption is straight sugar. We take it for granted; it is an accepted part of our daily routine. Yet, our primitive ancestors never saw or tasted refined sugar. It is an artifact of civilization.

In ancient times the Chinese called the juice of the sugarcane "stone honey"; the Greeks, "Indian salt" or "honey without bees"; the Romans, "saccharum." But in India where it originated, sugarcane was simply "khanda." The native populace chewed cane for sweetness and extracted the juice to spread on bread or pottage. Eventually they pressed the cane and drank the juice in much the way native Americans tapped maple trees. "Khanda" juice was highly perishable and would not keep without fermenting, so it had to be imbibed quickly after squeezing.

After Alexander the Great invaded India, sugarcane was brought back to Greece and Rome in tiny quantities. It was an expensive luxury restricted to the banquet tables of the very rich.

The physicians of ancient Persia are credited with developing a process of solidifying and refining the juice of the cane into a solid form. This new refined sugar was used medicinally as a sedative though—ironic when you consider how often it has been characterized as an energy food. Possibly its reputation as a sedative was due to the lowering of blood sugar after the initial energy rush, which acts to sedate the body.

Because it prolonged sugar's freshness before fermentation set in, this new discovery facilitated large-scale transportation and trade. Sugar became a leading commodity in the highly competitive world market.

The Sweet Tooth Fairy also took her toll on many Crusaders who, as they crossed the Middle East, wanted only to languish in the field, their bellies bloated with cane juice and sugar candy. And some European rulers suspected that their ambassadors to Egypt were being corrupted by the sweet-tooth habit with bribes of costly sugar.

When Christian conquerors discovered it was easier to plant the sugarcane at home than to import it, plantations sprouted up across Morea, Malta, and Sicily. Of more than twenty million Africans captured as slaves, over two-thirds were used to grow sugar.

Sugar and slavery were mostly a Portuguese monopoly, but Spain did not fall far behind with its sugarcane fields in Granada and Andalusia. At the suggestion of Queen Isabella, Christopher Columbus brought chunks of sugarcane on his second voyage to the New World and encouraged the building of plantations in the West Indies. While the rest of Europe was executing heretics and witches, the Portuguese were sending their condemned criminals to colonize South America and populate the sugarcane fields.

The development of sugar as a commercial product became one of the most profound influences on the Western world, as the Portuguese and Spanish empires rose to never-seen heights of opulence and power. When the British came to drive out the Spaniards, they took over the sugar plantations and slave trade in the Caribbean islands to ferment sugar into rum. The rum was traded to North American Indians for furs, which were shipped back to Europe and sold for a small fortune. From slaves to sugar to demon rum to furs to profit, it was an avaricious circle that would have made the Sweet Tooth Fairy proud.

Meanwhile, some of the sugar was made into molasses and sold to the American colonies. So intensive was this trade that the sugarcane fields in the Caribbean were soon totally exhausted by the overplanting of crops.

Any country with sugar trade could boast of great wealth and national importance. Heads of governments and European royalty took their cut of the wealth amassed by sugar plantation owners, traders, shippers, and the like with all the corruption of organized crime. One could speculate that our Sugar Fairy held as much sway over world greed as the Devil.

Great Britain remained the center of the world's commerce, but soon France cut in on this lucrative trade and refined sugar became her most important export. When war broke out between Napoleon and England, the British imposed a naval blockade around all French ports receiving raw sugar stock.

Napoleon searched near and far for "that taste" to satisfy the cravings of his armies, finally exerting pressure on French scientists to find a substitute for cane sugar. In 1812, Benjamin Delessert found a way to process beets into sugar, for which Napoleon awarded him the Legion of Honor. Sugar beets were planted everywhere in France. An imperial factory was established for refining. In a matter of a few years France had produced eight million pounds of sugar from beets. Long before Napoleon invaded Russia, his armies were well stocked with quick-energy sugar rations.

By the outset of the nineteenth century, America had emerged from the wings to upstage the European sugar monopolizers. Three American inventions—the steam engine, a technique for producing charcoal from animal bones, and the vacuum pan—led to the advent of white commercial sugar. The United States built giant refineries and colonized Cuba to produce the raw stock necessary for production.

From then on, the world of sugar would never be the same. This major breakthrough opened up a whole new market, greatly expanding the competition and thus lowering the price of sugar worldwide. With the prices down, sugar became affordable to all—a common staple in kitchens all across the globe.

While there were no more kings to grab their cut of the sugar business, the U.S. government started receiving very lucrative taxes. Cuban sugar bound for American factories accounted for 20 percent of the total federal revenue from import duty. We soon outdistanced every other nation in sugar production *and* its use—over *one-fifth* of the world's supply of sugar.

Today, sugar can be grown in the temperate zones as well as the tropics. The common man can easily afford it, and its consumption has spread far beyond the simple "khanda" of ancient India.

Given the unbelievable sugar commodity network throughout the world at present, manufacturers are selling us sugar whether we want it or not. Law requires that sugar be refined before it is sold—not necessarily an improvement. The sugar juice is pressed out of the cane, purified, filtered, boiled, centrifuged, and crystallized—then rammed down our throats in the form of additives.

So how is the constant use of this relatively new product affecting the human condition from generation to generation? Are our bodies being asked to make an evolutionary adaptive change to a new form of food intake? What is this stuff actually *doing* to our physical make-up?

Undeniably, emotions are a major trigger to cravings and hunger. A close second are triggers from advertising. The most susceptible individuals are those who overreact to sensory stimulation, such as those with candidiasis and allergic addictions. These two groups represent an enormous market for the food industry.

How can you resist? There is absolutely nothing you can do about the sugar in your environment. The billions spent on foods each year provide a healthy fund for hiring lobbyists to make sure nothing changes in current trends of merchandising. So forget the environmental factors. You can only change yourself. You now have one big advantage. The methods in this book will, in fact, neutralize the irresistible urges that overwhelm you. With your strength back, you can blunt their efforts to keep you addicted.

PART SIX

Resources

CHAPTER SIXTEEN

Getting Help

To gain maximum benefit from this book and to most effectively control your cravings, keep the following thoughts in mind.

1. You're unique

At first glance, our overall appearance is the same, but on closer inspection, there are countless differences between individuals. Our internal biochemical-physical makeup is unique also, for no two organisms are exactly alike.

The nutrients that block cravings will differ from one person to the next. You must search for your own special formula by changing the supplements until they're effective. How many times have you heard people say, "Oh, I tried that and it didn't work." But when you inquired how many times they tried, you were told, "Oh, once or twice."

Some people act as though they're helpless; they make a pitifully small effort and then quit if there's no one to encourage them. I hope *you* are going to do a lot better than that.

2. Circumstances are unique, too

Was there ever a time in your life when one event was identical to another? Of course not. Sometimes we think we experience *déjà vu*, but life doesn't actually repeat itself.

A formula that works well at one time may not succeed at another. With all of the suggestions found in this book, you'll have enough to work with in case you become tolerant to one set of supplements.

3. Time marches on

The human shape is quite plastic. It changes over the years. First we grow in height and girth, then we grow forward with the middle-age spread (unless we're careful), and finally we grow shorter with advanced age. If we suffer glandular disease, we may change in other ways. Hormones determine the shape of our bodies, also, and as hormone balance changes, so do we.

Our body chemistry balance too is subject to fluctuation. These patterns lead to new responses to nutrients. From time to time you may need to recompute your set of supplements.

4. A rose is a rose, but all cravings are not the same

As you can see by reading the chapter titles, there are dozens of causes for cravings; both triggers and functional changes motivate the urge to eat a particular food. Now that cravings are out of the closet and research is dealing with the problem, I think we'll see a lot of valuable material forthcoming. This may not sit well with the food industry, but we can't please everyone.

5. No one is immune

Old or young, fat or thin, tall or short, anyone can crave. Some do it daily, some crave only at particular times of the day, others at certain times of the month. Some cravings only begin after a person has been ill, while others strike at middle age. I think eventually, as research expands, classifications will become more refined.

6. Cravings can be the symptom of candidiasis

A craving can be the symptom of a mild imbalance of homeostasis, when things get slightly off kilter. But it can also indicate serious disease such as candidiasis. If you suspect that you suffer from it, you may need professional help. You might get in touch with the organizations listed in this chapter or seek additional consultation.

7. Cravings can be a symptom of allergy

Most food allergies can be self-managed if they are not too intense. However, there is a type called a fixed allergy, a permanent nonacquired allergy that will not respond to self-treatment. You'll have no choice but to seek professional help if this is the case.

8. Cravings: The serious side

Cravings and excessive hunger can be a sign of serious disease. Excessive hunger can be a problem to obese individuals, but it can also be caused by an overactive thyroid (hyperthyroidism) or by diabetes. Excessive thirst can be caused by diabetes, kidney disease, or excessive use of diuretics ("water pills"). Coffee or alcohol in excess may also dehydrate the body and cause severe thirst (polydipsia). If for any reason you suspect you may have one of these, or other problems, *see your physician before using any of the supplements listed in this book.*

9. *You can do it*

Nutritional supplements are highly effective in blocking cravings. With practice you can become an expert. Controlling cravings doesn't mean you need an iron will; mostly it means using your head to figure out what you need. It also means spending a little time on trial and error. My experience has shown that most people can find an effective remedy if they are patient.

There are drugs that will also bring results. If you can't control cravings nutritionally, you might seek the cooperation of a physician. Don't expect to walk into a doctor's office and receive a prescription without the physician's evaluation. Doctors aren't pharmacists; they must decide whether it's wise or unwise to use medications for a particular ailment. They also require assurances that drugs won't be abused. The overuse of drugs is a major problem in today's society, and some of the drugs used to control cravings can fall into this category.

WHERE TO SEEK HELP

If you have decided to seek professional help, where do you look?

Your local Yellow Pages

Look under *Physicians and Surgeons—M.D.* There will be a listing in alphabetical order, followed by specialty listings. Also look under *Nutrition* or *Preventive Medicine*. Be sure you make sufficient inquiries on the phone before booking an appointment.

Nutritionists

Many good nutritionists can be of benefit. Those in private practice usually dispense knowledgeable diet information.

Though nutritionists offer valuable services, remember that they can't write prescriptions, so if you need medication, consult a physician.

Health food stores

You're sure to get advice here, but don't take it blindly. Store owners are often well informed, but counter clerks may be inexperienced. Don't assume that because someone works in a health food store that person has knowledge of nutrition.

Your local druggist

Pharmacists can assist you in finding the products you are looking for. Some are well versed in nutrition, but if not, they may help you find a doctor who specializes in nutritional medicine.

Professional organizations concerned with candidiasis and allergy addictions

Doctors who belong to the organizations listed here have usually attended seminars and conferences about allergic addictions and candidiasis. They read the journals related to clinical ecology and allergy and have experience with such patients. Not all the members of these organizations have an interest in these subjects, so ask questions when you contact member doctors.

Human Ecology Action
League
505 N. Lakeshore Dr.
#6505
Chicago, IL 60611

American Academy of
Environmental Medicine
P.O. Box 16106
Denver, CO 80216

American Society of
  Bariatric Physicians
7430 E. Coley #210
Englewood, CO 80111
1-800-621-8385, Ext. 427

American Society of
  Bariatric Surgeons
625 Post Street #639
San Francisco, CA 94109

Academy of Orthomolecular
  Psychiatry
1691 Northern Boulevard
Manhasset, NY 11031

International College of
  Applied Nutrition
P.O. Box 286
La Habra, CA 90631

Price Pottenger Foundation
P.O. Box 2614
La Mesa, CA 92041

American Academy of
  Medical Preventics
6151 West Century
  Boulevard
Los Angeles, CA 90045

The Orthomolecular
  Medical Society
6151 West Century
  Boulevard
Los Angeles, CA 90045

International Academy of
  Preventive Medicine
P.O. Box 25276
Shawnee Mission, KS
  66225

American Academy of
  Otolaryngic Allergy
1101 Vermont Avenue
  N.W. #302
Washington, DC 20005

Other information sources:

Access to Nutritional Data
P.O. Box 52
Ashby, MA 01431

Human Ecology Action
  League (H.E.A.L.)
7330 N. Rojers Avenue
Chicago, IL 60626

Center for Science in the
  Public Interest
1501 16th Street N.W.
Washington, DC 20036

Gale Neilson
P.O. Box 2719
Castro Valley, CA 94546
415-582-2179

Organizations that deal with PMS:

National PMS Society
P.O. Box 11467
Durham, NC 27703

PMS Action Inc.
P.O. Box 9326
Madison, WI 53715

Family and Teen Health
   Services
Green County Memorial
   Hospital
Waynesburg, PA 15370

PMS Research Foundation
P.O. Box 14574
Las Vegas, NV 89114

PMS Community Awareness
1914 Chandler Lane
Columbus, IN 47203

PMS Center
9201 Sunset Boulevard
Los Angeles, CA 90069

PMS Treatment Center
150 N. Santa Anita
Arcadia, CA 91006

PMS Connection
Women's Medical Center
5985 W. Pico Boulevard
Los Angeles, CA 90035

Dr. Michelle Harrison
763 Massachusetts Avenue
Cambridge, MA 02139

Premenstrual Syndrome
   Consultants of Colorado
6415 W. 44th
Wheatridge, CO 80033

PMS Medical Group
140 West End Avenue
New York, NY 10023

Selecting a doctor when you need medical assistance

Family physician. It might be difficult for patients with excessive hunger, excessive cravings, or any of the symptoms listed in this book to find help from a family physician. Unfortunately, physicians resist patients' demands for help with a problem the doctor may not be familiar with. If you need help with a food allergy or suspected candidiasis infection, the family doctor will usually not be helpful.

Psychiatrists and psychologists. It might seem strange to be referred to a psychiatrist for help with a food allergy or candidiasis. It is not strange at all. Psychiatrists often are at the forefront of innovation. Psychiatric assistance may be necessary in addition to medical care if these problems have existed for a long time. Severe depression or even thoughts of suicide occur in some patients with long-term candidiasis. In such a case the acute symptoms must be treated before the chronic symptoms are treated.

Female physicians. Women are frequently more open-minded than men to new ideas—at least it seems so in medicine. A female physician is often the right person to see, especially if she is aware of food allergies and candidiasis.

Weight control doctors. Only a few are knowledgeable regarding food allergies and cravings. Check with them before you make your appointment.

Allergists and clinical ecologists. Most doctors in this group have spent a good deal of their own time and money learning this specialty. They fully understand all phases of allergy and food addiction. Further, they have probably seen dozens of cases of candidiasis. They know food allergy very well. But there is just one problem. There are too many people with health problems and too few clinical ecologists. Most doctors in this group have backgrounds in allergy, internal medicine, or psychiatry and are well equipped to assist you.

SAMPLE PERSONAL CRAVINGS DIARY

Day One

Time of Craving	Time of Supplement	Time Relief Felt	Time Cravings Returned	Supplements to Be Used Today
8 A.M.				
9 A.M.				
10 A.M.				
11 A.M.				
12 noon				
1 P.M.				
2 P.M.				
3 P.M.				
4 P.M.				
5 P.M.				
6 P.M.				
7 P.M.				
8 P.M.				
9 P.M.				
10 P.M.				
11 P.M.				

Directions: (1) Record supplements to be used for the day in upper right corner. (2) Record time when supplement is taken. (3) Record time relief from craving is felt. (4) Record time craving returns. (5) Continue recording throughout the day. (6) If relief from cravings lasts longer than 4 hours, take supplement less frequently. (7) When you arrive at a schedule that works, you may discontinue diary. (8) If selected formula does not work, set up a new one the following day. (9) Select from substances suggested and change the formula each day until you arrive at your individual, personalized regime.

SAMPLE PERSONAL CRAVINGS DIARY

Day Two

Time of Craving	Time of Supplement	Time Relief Felt	Time Cravings Returned	Supplements to Be Used Today
8 A.M.				
9 A.M.				
10 A.M.				
11 A.M.				
12 noon				
1 P.M.				
2 P.M.				
3 P.M.				
4 P.M.				
5 P.M.				
6 P.M.				
7 P.M.				
8 P.M.				
9 P.M.				
10 P.M.				
11 P.M.				

Directions: (1) Record supplements to be used for the day in upper right corner. (2) Record time when supplement is taken. (3) Record time relief from craving is felt. (4) Record time craving returns. (5) Continue recording throughout the day. (6) If relief from cravings lasts longer than 4 hours, take supplement less frequently. (7) When you arrive at a schedule that works, you may discontinue diary. (8) If selected formula does not work, set up a new one the following day. (9) Select from substances suggested and change the formula each day until you arrive at your individual, personalized regime.

SAMPLE PERSONAL CRAVINGS DIARY

Day Three

Time of Craving	Time of Supplement	Time Relief Felt	Time Cravings Returned	Supplements to Be Used Today
8 A.M.				
9 A.M.				
10 A.M.				
11 A.M.				
12 noon				
1 P.M.				
2 P.M.				
3 P.M.				
4 P.M.				
5 P.M.				
6 P.M.				
7 P.M.				
8 P.M.				
9 P.M.				
10 P.M.				
11 P.M.				

Directions: (1) Record supplements to be used for the day in upper right corner. (2) Record time when supplement is taken. (3) Record time relief from craving is felt. (4) Record time craving returns. (5) Continue recording throughout the day. (6) If relief from cravings lasts longer than 4 hours, take supplement less frequently. (7) When you arrive at a schedule that works, you may discontinue diary. (8) If selected formula does not work, set up a new one the following day. (9) Select from substances suggested and change the formula each day until you arrive at your individual, personalized regime.

SAMPLE PERSONAL CRAVINGS DIARY

Day Four

Time of Craving	Time of Supplement	Time Relief Felt	Time Cravings Returned	Supplements to Be Used Today
8 A.M.				
9 A.M.				
10 A.M.				
11 A.M.				
12 noon				
1 P.M.				
2 P.M.				
3 P.M.				
4 P.M.				
5 P.M.				
6 P.M.				
7 P.M.				
8 P.M.				
9 P.M.				
10 P.M.				
11 P.M.				

Directions: (1) Record supplements to be used for the day in upper right corner. (2) Record time when supplement is taken. (3) Record time relief from craving is felt. (4) Record time craving returns. (5) Continue recording throughout the day. (6) If relief from cravings lasts longer than 4 hours, take supplement less frequently. (7) When you arrive at a schedule that works, you may discontinue diary. (8) If selected formula does not work, set up a new one the following day. (9) Select from substances suggested and change the formula each day until you arrive at your individual, personalized regime.

SAMPLE PERSONAL CRAVINGS DIARY

Day Five

Time of Craving	Time of Supplement	Time Relief Felt	Time Cravings Returned	Supplements to Be Used Today
8 A.M.				
9 A.M.				
10 A.M.				
11 A.M.				
12 noon				
1 P.M.				
2 P.M.				
3 P.M.				
4 P.M.				
5 P.M.				
6 P.M.				
7 P.M.				
8 P.M.				
9 P.M.				
10 P.M.				
11 P.M.				

Directions: (1) Record supplements to be used for the day in upper right corner. (2) Record time when supplement is taken. (3) Record time relief from craving is felt. (4) Record time craving returns. (5) Continue recording throughout the day. (6) If relief from cravings lasts longer than 4 hours, take supplement less frequently. (7) When you arrive at a schedule that works, you may discontinue diary. (8) If selected formula does not work, set up a new one the following day. (9) Select from substances suggested and change the formula each day until you arrive at your individual, personalized regime.

SAMPLE PERSONAL CRAVINGS DIARY

Day Six

Time of Craving	Time of Supplement	Time Relief Felt	Time Cravings Returned	Supplements to Be Used Today
8 A.M.				
9 A.M.				
10 A.M.				
11 A.M.				
12 noon				
1 P.M.				
2 P.M.				
3 P.M.				
4 P.M.				
5 P.M.				
6 P.M.				
7 P.M.				
8 P.M.				
9 P.M.				
10 P.M.				
11 P.M.				

Directions: (1) Record supplements to be used for the day in upper right corner. (2) Record time when supplement is taken. (3) Record time relief from craving is felt. (4) Record time craving returns. (5) Continue recording throughout the day. (6) If relief from cravings lasts longer than 4 hours, take supplement less frequently. (7) When you arrive at a schedule that works, you may discontinue diary. (8) If selected formula does not work, set up a new one the following day. (9) Select from substances suggested and change the formula each day until you arrive at your individual, personalized regime.

SAMPLE PERSONAL CRAVINGS DIARY

Day Seven

Time of Craving	Time of Supplement	Time Relief Felt	Time Cravings Returned	Supplements to Be Used Today
8 A.M.				
9 A.M.				
10 A.M.				
11 A.M.				
12 noon				
1 P.M.				
2 P.M.				
3 P.M.				
4 P.M.				
5 P.M.				
6 P.M.				
7 P.M.				
8 P.M.				
9 P.M.				
10 P.M.				
11 P.M.				

Directions: (1) Record supplements to be used for the day in upper right corner. (2) Record time when supplement is taken. (3) Record time relief from craving is felt. (4) Record time craving returns. (5) Continue recording throughout the day. (6) If relief from cravings lasts longer than 4 hours, take supplement less frequently. (7) When you arrive at a schedule that works, you may discontinue diary. (8) If selected formula does not work, set up a new one the following day. (9) Select from substances suggested and change the formula each day until you arrive at your individual, personalized regime.

REFERENCES

Abraham, G.E., and Lutran, M.M. "Serum and Red Cell Magnesium in Patients with Premenstrual Syndrome." *American Journal of Clinical Nutrition* 34. 1981.

Abrahamson, E.M., and Peget, A.W. *Body, Mind and Sugar.* New York: Avon, 1951.

Aillon, G.A. "Biochemistry of Affective Disorders." *Psychosomatics* 12. 1971.

Austen, K., Wasserman, S.I., and Goetzel, E.J. *Molecular and Biological Aspects of the Acute Allergic Reactions.* New York: Plenum, 1978.

Beisel, W. "Single Nutrient Effects on Immunological Functions." *JAMA* 245. 1981.

Bell, I.R. *Clinical Ecology.* Bolinas, California: Common Knowledge Press. 1982.

Bergel, F. *Homeostatic Regulators.* London: Ciba Foundation. 1969.

Bernhart, M., Gellhorn, E., and Rasmussen, A.T. "Experimental Contributions to the Problem of Consciousness." *Journal of Neurophysiology* 19. 1953.

Birch, G.G. *Sensory Properties of Foods.* London: Applied Science. 1977.

Bolton, S. "Caffeine. Its Effects, Uses and Abuses." *Journal of Applied Nutrition* 33. 1981.

Booth, D.A. *Hunger Models, Computable Theory of Feeding Control*. New York: Academic Press. 1978.

Boyd, E.M. *Toxicity of Pure Foods*. Cleveland: CRC Press. 1973.

Brin, M., and Iversen, L. "Chemistry of the Brain." *Scientific American*. June 1980.

Cameron, E., and Pauling, L. *Cancer and Vitamin C*. New York: W.W. Norton, 1979.

Casper, R.C. "Bulimia and Diet." *Archives of General Psychiatry*. 1980.

Cheraskin, E., Ringsdorf, W.M., and Brescher, A. *Psychodietetics*. New York: Harper & Row. 1983.

Chernin, R. *The Obsession: Reflections on the Tyranny of Slenderness*. New York: Harper & Row. 1981.

Coombs, R.A., and Gell, P.G.H. *Clinical Aspects of Immunology*. Oxford: Blackwell. 1968.

Costa, E., and Trabucchi, M. *The Endorphins*. New York: Raven Press.

Crook, William G. *Tracking Down Hidden Food Allergies*. Jackson, Tennessee: Professional Books. 1978.

———. *The Yeast Connection*. Jackson, Tennessee: Professional Books. 1983.

Cullen, J.W., and Scarborough, B.B. "Effects of a Preoperative Sugar Preference on Bar Pressing for Salt by the Adrenolectomized Rat." *Journal of Comparative Physiology and Psychology* 67. 1969.

Dahi, L.K. "Salt and Hypertension." *American Journal of Clinical Nutrition* 25. 1972.

Dalton, Katharine. *Once a Month*. Claremont, California: Hunter House. 1979.

Davis, P. "Nutrition Needs and Biochemical Diversity." *Medical Applications of Clinical Nutrition*. New Canaan, Connecticut: Keats. 1983.

Denton, Derek. *The Hunger for Salt*. New York: Springer. 1982.

D'Orban, P.T. "Premenstrual Syndrome: A Disease of the Mind." *Lancet*. December 1981.

Dufty, W. *Sugar Blues*. Denver, Colorado: Nutri Books Corp. 1982.

Eddy, Walter H. *Vitaminology*. Baltimore: Williams & Wilkins, 1949.

Ellis, A. *Reason and Emotion in Psychotherapy*. New York: Lyle Stewart. 1962.

Faelten, S. *The Allergy Self-Help Book*. Emmaus, Pennsylvania: Rodale Press. 1970

Faust, I.M. *The Body Weight Regulatory System*. New York: Raven Press. 1981.

Feingold, H. *Why Your Child Is Hyperactive*. New York: Random House. 1975.

Ferguson, A., and Strobel, S. "Immunology and Physiology of Digestion." *In:* Lessof, M. H. (Ed.) *Clinical Reactions to Food*. New York: John Wiley & Sons. 1983.

Forbes, G.B. "Is Obesity a Genetic Disease?" *Contemporary Nutrition* No. 8. 1981.

Forman, R. *How to Control Your Allergies*. New York: Larchmont Books. 1979.

Fox, J. "Scientists Face Explosion of Brain Compounds." *Chemical and Engineering News*. November 1979.

Fredericks, C. *Psycho Nutrition*. New York: Grosset & Dunlop. 1976.

Garrow, J.S. *Energy Balance and Obesity in Man*. New York: Elsevier. 1978.

Geiselman, P.L., and Norin, D. "Sugar Infusion Can Enhance Feeding." *Science* 213. 1982.

Glass, A.R., Burman, K.D., and Boehm, T.M. "Endocrine Function in Obesity." *Metabolism* 30. 1981.

Goldfried, M.R., and Goldfried, A.P. *Helping People Change*. New York: Pergamon Press. 1980.

Golos, N., Goldbitz, F., and Leighton, F. *Coping with Your Allergies*. New York: Simon and Schuster. 1979.

Goodall, J. "Feeding Behavior of Wild Chimpanzees, A Preliminary Report." *Symposia of the Zoological Society of London*, Vol. 10, no. 39. 1963.

Gray, J. *The Psychology of Fear and Stress*. McGraw-Hill: New York. 1971.

Green, R.S., and Rau, J.H. *Anorexia Nervosa*. New York: Raven Press. 1977.

Gross, M. *The Psychological Society*. New York: Simon and Schuster. 1978.

Hall, R.H. *Food for Naught*. New York: Harper & Row. 1977.

Hamburg, D.A. "Health and Behavior." *Science* 213. 1982.

Hare, F. *The Food Factor in Disease*. London: Green and Co. 1905.

Hemmings, W. *Food Antigens and the Gut*. Lancaster Press. 1979.

Hoffer, Myron A. *Roots of Human Behavior*. San Francisco: W.H. Freeman. 1981.

Hunter, B.T. *The Great Nutritional Robbery*. New York: Scribners. 1978.

Jarvis, D.C. *Arthritis and Folk Medicine*. New York: Fawcett. 1960.

————. *Folk Medicine*. New York: Henry Holt & Company. 1958.

Klopf, H.A. *The Hedonistic Neuron*. San Francisco, California: Hemisphere. 1982.

Kolata, G. "Brain Receptors for Appetite Discovered." *Science* 218. 1982.

Lansky, V. *The Taming of the C.A.N.D.Y. Monster*. Wayzatn, Minnesota: Meadowbrook Press. 1978.

Lasky, M.S. *The Complete Junk Food Book*. New York: McGraw-Hill. 1977.

Lesser, M. *Nutrition and Vitamin Therapy*. New York: Grove Press. 1980.

Levenkron, S. *The Best Little Girl in the World*. New York: Warner Books. 1978.

Levine, S. *Antioxidant Biochemical Adaptation*. San Leandro, California: Biocurrents Research Corp. 1984.

Levitt, T. *Marketing for Business Growth*. New York: McGraw-Hill. 1969.

Lindner, R. *The Fifty-Minute Hour*. New York: Reinhart. 1954.

Luce, Gay. *Body Time*. New York: Pantheon Books. 1971.

Mackomess, R. *Eating Dangerously: The Hazards of Hidden Allergies*. New York: Harcourt Brace Jovanovich. 1976.

Magovin, H.W. *The Walking Brain*. Springfield, Illinois: Charles C Thomas. 1963.

McDonald, R. "Effect of Visible Light Waves on Arthritis Pains." *International Journal of Biosocial Research*. 1982.

Maller, Owen. "Specific Appetite." *In:* Kare, M.R., and Maller, O. (Eds.) *The Chemical Senses and Nutrition.* Baltimore: John Hopkins Press. 1967.

Mandell, M., and Scanlon, L. *Dr. Mandell's Five-Day Allergy Relief System.* New York: Pocket Books. 1979.

Miller, J. *Food Allergy.* Springfield, Illinois: Charles C. Thomas. 1972.

Millman, M. *Such a Pretty Face: Being Fat in America.* New York: Berkley Books. 1980.

Mitchell, James E., et al. "The Bulimic Syndrome in Normal Weight Individuals: A Review." *International Journal of Eating Disorders.* Winter (1981).

Monroe, J., and Brostoff, J. "Food Allergy in Migraine." *Lancet.* July 1980.

Myers, K. "Morphological Changes in the Adrenal Glands of Wild Rabbits." *Nature* 213:147.

Newbolt, H.L. *Mega Nutrients for Your Nerves.* New York: Wyden Books. 1978.

Norvin, D. *Hunger, Basic Mechanisms and Clinical Implications.* New York: Raven Press. 1976.

Orbach, S. *Fat Is a Feminist Issue.* New York: Berkley Books. 1978.

Ott, J. Berkley, *Light and Health.* New York: Bantam. 1977.

Page, L., and Friend, B. "The Changing U.S. Diet." *Bioscience* 28. 1978.

Perls, F. *Ego, Hunger and Aggression.* New York: Random House. 1969.

Philpott, W.H., and Kalita, B.K. *Brain Allergies.* New Canaan, Connecticut: Keats. 1980.

Pike, R., and Brown, M. "Nutrition—An Integrated Approach." New York: John Wiley & Sons. 1984.

Rapp, D.J. *Allergies and the Hyperactive Child.* New York: Sovereign. 1979.

———. *Allergies and Your Family.* New York: Sterling. 1981.

Randolph, T.G. *Human Ecology and Susceptibility to the Chemical Environment.* Springfield, Illinois: Charles C. Thomas. 1962.

———, and Moss, R.W. *An Alternative Approach to Allergies.* New York: Lippincott & Crowell. 1979.

Richter, C.P., and Eckert, J.F. "Mineral Metabolism of Adrenalectomized Rats Studied by the Appetite Method." *Endocrinology* 22. 1938.

Rowe, Albert H., and Rowe, Albert Jr. *Food Allergy, Its Manifestations and Control and the Elimination Diet.* Springfield, Illinois: Charles C. Thomas. 1972.

Schauss, A. *Diet, Crime and Delinquency.* Berkeley, California: Parker House. 1981.

Schroeder, H.A. *Trace Elements and Man.* Old Greenwich, Connecticut: Devin-Adair. 1973.

Selye, H. *Stress.* Montreal, Canada: Acta, Inc. 1950.

Shahied, I. *Biochemistry of Foods and Biocatalysts.* New York: Vantage Press. 1977.

Sheinkin, D., Schacter, M., and Hutton, R. *Food, Mind and Mood.* New York: Warner Books. 1980.

Sloan, S. *Nutritional Parenting.* New Canaan, Connecticut: Keats. 1982.

Smith, L.H. *Foods for Healthy Kids.* New York: McGraw-Hill. 1981.

Sochar, E. *Topics in Psychoendocrinology.* New York: Grune & Stratton. 1975.

Spiller, G.A. *Nutritional Pharmacology.* New York: Alan Liss. 1982.

Stuart, Richard B., and Davis, Barbara. *Slim Chance in a Fat World—Behavorial Control of Obesity.* Champaign, Illinois: Research Press. 1972.

Thompson, C.J. *Controls of Eating.* Jamaica, New York: Spectrum Publications. 1980.

Vincent, L.S. *Competing with the Sylph.* Kansas City: Andrews & McNeel. 1979.

Weiss, J.M., Stone, E.A., and Harrell, N. "Coping Behavior and Brain Norepinephrine Level in Rats." *Journal of Comparative and Physiological Psychology* 72. 1970.

Wharton, G.W. "An Ecological Study of the Kouprey." Institute of Science and Technology, Manila (Monograph No. 5).

Whatmore, G.B. *Tension in Medicine.* Springfield, Illinois: Charles C. Thomas. 1967.

———, and Kohli, D.R. "Dysponesis. A Neurophysiologic

Factor in Functional Disorders." *Behavioral Science* 13. 1968.

————, and Kohli, D.R. *The Physiopathology and Treatment of Functional Disorders.* New York: Grune & Stratton. 1974.

Wilkins, L., and Richter, C.P. "A Great Craving for Salt by a Child with Corticoadrenal Insufficiency. *Journal of the American Medical Association* 114. 1940.

Williams, J. "Iron Deficiency Treatment." *Western Journal of Medicine.* February 1981.

Williams, R.J. *Nutrition against Disease.* New York: Bantam Books. 1973.

Wolpe, J. *The Practice of Behavioral Therapy.* New York: Pergamon Press. 1969.

Wunderlich, R.C. *Sugar and Your Health.* St. Petersburg, Florida: Good Health. 1982.

Wunderlich, R., and Kolita, D. Candidia *and the Human Condition.* New Canaan, Connecticut: Keats. 1984.

Wurtman, J.J., and Zeisel, S.H. "Carbohydrate Cravings in Obese People." *International Journal of Eating Disorders.* February 1982.

Wurtman, R.J. "Nutrients That Modify Brain Functions." *Scientific American.* June 1982.

Young, J.K. "A Possible Neuroendocrine Basis of Two Clinical Syndromes: Anorexia Nervosa, and the Klein-Levin Syndrome. *Physiological Psychology* 3. 1975.

Zamm, A.V., and Gannon, R. *Why Your House May Endanger Your Health.* New York: Simon and Schuster. 1980.

INDEX